Keto for Cancer

A Practical Guide to a Healthful and Natural Approach to Stopping and Slowing Cancer Growth with Metabolic Recovery

By Mark Arizona

Table of Contents

Introduction
Chapter 1: The Nature of the Illness
  What is Cancer?
  Metastasis: How Cancer Travels and Grows
  Metabolic Reasons for Cancer
  Autoimmune Disorders and Cancer
  Glucose Ketone Index
Chapter 2: The Keto-Cancer Relationship
  Glucose and Cancer Cell Proliferation
  Glucose and Glutamine as Cancer Cell Food
  The Problem with the Metabolism of Glucose
Chapter 3: Ketosis
  What is Ketosis?
  How do I Get into Ketosis?
  What Things Could Take Me Out of Ketosis?
  Is Ketosis Vital to Keto and to Fighting Cancer?
  What is Ketoacidosis and How do I Avoid it?
Chapter 4: A Word on Fasting
  What is Intermittent Fasting?
  How does Intermittent Fasting Affect Cancer Cells?
  The Benefits of Intermittent Fasting
  The Types of Fasting
    The 12/12 Fast
    The 16/8 Fast
    The 20/4 Fast
    5:2 Day Fasting

Chapter 5: The Keto Essentials
  Important Things to Remember
  Medical Fitness
  The Right Things to Eat
  The Wrong Things to Eat
  Detoxifying Your Kitchen
Chapter 6: How Keto Changes Your Metabolism
  Glucose Dependent Metabolism
  Fat Dependent Metabolism
  What are Macronutrients?
  The Right Macro Balance
  How to Track Macros
Chapter 7: FAQ
Chapter 8: Tips & Tricks for Sticking to Keto
Chapter 9: Keto Breakfast Recipes
  Taco Breakfast Skillet
  Keto Breakfast Sandwich
  Oatlessmeal
  Pulled Pork Hash
Chapter 10: Keto Lunch Recipes
  Shredded Beef
  Dairy-Free Butter Chicken
  Salmon Salad
  Chicken Avocado Salad
Chapter 11: Keto Dinner Recipes
  White Chicken Chili
  Spaghetti Squash with Bacon Blue Cheese
  Spinach Artichoke Chicken

    Korean Beef over Cauliflower Rice
Chapter 12: Keto Snack Recipes
    Parmesan Zucchini Fries
    Zesty Ranch Cauliflower Crisps
    Peanut Butter Bars
    Lemon Poppy Seed Muffins
Chapter 13: Keto Dessert Recipes
    Chewy Chocolate Cookies
    Berry Cheesecake Bars
    Coconut Lime Bars
    Strawberry Ice Cream
Conclusion
Resources

Introduction

Congratulations on purchasing *Keto for Cancer: A Practical Guide to a Healthful and Natural Approach to Stopping and Slowing Cancer Growth with Metabolic Recovery* and thank you for doing so.

If you've purchased this book, then it probably means that you have a concern about the subject of cancer, that you know there is more to it than is readily apparent, and that you have confidence in your body's natural ability to combat and recover from illnesses. The state of healthcare in certain countries and the position of large pharmaceutical companies makes it hard to be able to take an impartial, unbiased, and completely informed look at the subject. There are simply too many sources of information in today's modern age that completely conflict with one another.

If you're anything like the vast majority of adults in today's world, you're simply trying to make the best life possible for yourself and for the people that you love, and you want to get the best possible outcome for your treatment and for your life in general. That is only natural and you're doing the right thing by looking to other informative sources to understand all the information that is currently available on the subject of the body, its ability to fight off cancer, its ability to heal, and how it can work in tandem with recent medical advances to rid your body of harmful diseases without sacrificing your long-term health and vitality.

At the moment when the diagnosis is given, the patient and the family immediately go into a panic, wondering what they can do to fight the illness, wondering how much it's going to cost, wondering how long it's going to take to recover, wondering if they're going to lose the person that's dear to them, and so much more. That is only natural, considering the gravity of such a diagnosis. However, there are a lot of things to know right at the point of diagnosis so you can make sure that the course of treatment being chosen is the right one for you, for your family, and to contribute to the longest, most ideal life for you.

With so much information available on the internet today, it's kind of a wonder anyone is able to keep their head above water, isn't it? Luckily for you, this book holds the perfect balance of answers about your body's abilities to heal and how those abilities can work *with* your medical treatment for the best possible outcome. This book lays out everything you need to know about cancer, about how it works in the body, about how it's formed, about what kills it, and about what you can actually do to fight off this illness and to prolong your life.

This book is one of the most valuable tools you will find in helping you to curate the perfect path to wellness for yourself, as it perfectly blends the medical advances you need with the health information that will keep you feeling your best throughout treatment.

More and more doctors across the world are beginning to acknowledge the connections between the foods that we eat and the diseases we suffer from. As they're doing so, they're finding that vital changes to the dietary habits of each patient have vastly aided in the healing and recovery processes for each patient they've seen!

There are countless ailments that are prevalent today solely because of the poor diets of millions of patients. If we're able to identify the things that make a "poor diet," and we're able to point out the places in which you can improve your intake and your overall health, then your body will gain more and more ground in the fight against harmful diseases, growths, and illnesses that can drastically shorten one's lifetime.

I know how incredibly important family is and I know how incredibly vital it is to be here as long as you possibly can for the people you love. That is why I've taken it upon myself to sift through all the research, to go through all the complex medical explanations of everything and to bring you a completely unbiased answer about how you can completely rehabilitate your body, recover from the ravages of cancer, and come back feeling better than you did before your diagnosis!

There are millions of people who have experienced life-changing improvements when they started paying attention to the things they're putting into their bodies and when they started to make a conscious decision to eat only the foods that took them toward greater, better health. By taking control of the foods you eat, you're taking control of the things that you're putting into your body that could potentially be setting you back on your goals for health and vitality. When you can monitor the foods you're eating and when you can be certain that you're not putting harmful chemicals, pesticides, preservatives, additives, and fillers into your diet, you can have a greater sense of security about your future.

It's that security that the millions of people diagnosed with cancer all over the globe need. Feeling like you're in the driver's seat and like you have a definite say in your own future can make all the difference when you're undergoing treatment for cancer, whatever type it may be.

In this book, you will learn about what cancer is, what causes it, what correlation there is between the foods you eat and the propagation and reduction of the illness. You will learn about the connections between cancer, diet, and autoimmune diseases and you will learn how to use that connection to your advantage.

The first months after diagnosis are critical and what you do during that time could drastically affect the outcome of your treatment. By taking this step to make the best possible moves in the beginning stages of your treatment, you are taking control, putting yourself in an active role in your treatment, and you are making sure that your chances are as good as they can possibly be with the help of your doctor.

It is my promise to you that you will find information in this book that will prove vital to you during your fight with cancer, whether you're personally diagnosed or whether it's someone who is close to you. The information in this book provides a clear insight into the science behind the disease and its cure. Focus on the answers with scientific background and basis and focus on the information your doctor gives you, and you will get through this like a champion.

I have made every effort possible to thoroughly research the points being relayed in this book and I have given it my all to ensure that the best information is laid here at your fingertips and explained in a way that is approachable, digestible, understandable, and applicable.

Acting quickly when the diagnosis is given is crucial and deciding on the route for treatment is vital. By understanding as much as you can, as early as you can, you're going into this fight far more prepared than some others have been. Don't wait to continue reading, as it could put you at somewhat of a disadvantage. Don't let yourself lose any ground in this fight against this illness. You can make it through this fight with help from your body and your doctor. With the right information, you'll even make it look easy to everyone around you!

Don't delay and don't risk your symptoms and suffering getting any worse. Continue reading on to the next chapter now so you can live a long and healthy life, on your own terms!

CHAPTER 1: THE NATURE OF THE ILLNESS

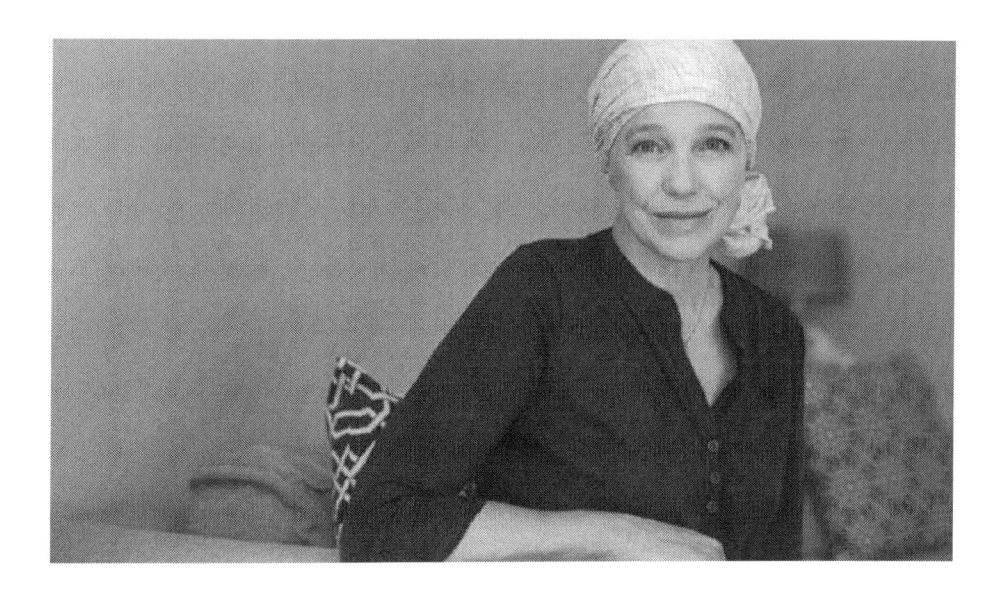

What is Cancer?

Cancer is an illness that can begin just about anywhere in the body and which can spread through the uncontrolled separation and reproduction of affected cells. These cancerous cells will overtake (or attempt to overtake) the other, healthy cells around them. Because cells are vital to the processes within the body and because the reproduction of healthy cells is what allows us to continue being healthy, the growth of cancer cells can be quite damaging.

One of the things it's important to know about cancer and the way in which it works is that it is not one disease. Cancer is an umbrella term for a couple hundred various diseases that share this cellular behavior. All of these cancers have their own unique traits and behaviors, and as a result of this, they all have their own particular type of treatment that is ideal for them.

Cancers are alike in their basic construction and the way in which they spread. Healthy cells that are not affected by cancer will routinely divide and multiply in a very neat and structured way. With cancer cells, there isn't any rhyme or reason to their multiplication patterns, which means that acting fast is absolutely crucial when treating cancer. It can be very difficult to form any kind of projection or pattern the cancer will follow when growing, so the sooner it's removed from the body, the better.

However, there are some cancers that typically move at a different rate than others. While the rate may not be steady, the average speed might be slower than that of other cancers, which can help your doctor to know a little bit more about the most appropriate timeline to keep when treating you for your illness.

Cancer is a type of illness that requires a rather aggressive course of treatment from doctors who are familiar with the patterns of growth, with the things that stop it in its tracks, and vigilance on the part of the patient to reduce and mitigate risk factors that could make it more likely or more possible for cancer to grow again or to spread throughout the body.

We'll cover how cancer travels through the body in the next section of this chapter.

Metastasis: How Cancer Travels and Grows

Metastasis is the development of more malignant (infectious) growths in the body that are in a different location than the primary growth or the first one that was spotted. This means that if you have a cancerous growth in your right lung and the growth is then spotted in the left lung, that is a different part of the body and the cancer has reached metastasis or it has *metastasized*.

If cancer goes unchecked for too long and the cells are

given the chance to continue to grow, a cancer can reach metastasis. It is also possible for it to happen in spite of treatment in some unfortunate cases. It's impossible to be right 100% of the time, but oncologists and surgeons certainly try their best to keep this from happening.

The primary means of transport for cancerous cells to grow in other parts of the body are the lymphatic system and the bloodstream. If a cancerous cell makes its way into one of these internal superhighways, then it could end up in virtually any place in the body, making it that much harder to track down and remove from the body.

In many cases, once a cancer has reached metastatic levels, it can no longer be cured. There are some cases in which this is not true and there are cases of metastatic cancer that result in the recovery of the patient. Most doctors find it prudent to note, however, that this is not the norm and once cancer reaches metastasis, it's very difficult to come back from it.

As mentioned previously, cancer grows within the body by multiplying the cancerous cells at an uncontrolled rate. These cells will divide just as normal cells would, creating many more of themselves. Once your body holds a clump of cancerous cells, the other cells around it that are healthy are left to fight for the space they need in order to keep your body working properly. This is what gives cancer its symptoms and causes your body to react poorly to these cells that are produced in your body.

Metabolic Reasons for Cancer

In the past, cancer has only been regarded as a disease of proliferation, meaning that it's simply a disease that thrives on its own ability to multiply its cells within the body. However, as we get closer to the root causes of cancer, there are some signs to suggest that it could also be considered a metabolic disease. This is because the tumors that grow (the clumps of cancerous cells) will rework their own metabolic processes to facilitate continuous growth. This means that it's able to change the demands it has for fuel to keep on growing.

The types of things that cancer can feed on in order to grow can change over time in order to allow it to thrive. If the person who has cancer is eating a regular diet that is rich in carbohydrates, the body will sustain itself off of glucose, which is what your body will turn its food into. Glucose is the current fuel source of your body when you're not doing a ketogenic diet of any kind. Tumors have been known to consume and sustain off of glucose in the body.

It's from this conclusion that some have deduced that greatly reducing the amount of glucose in the body can help to "starve" the cancer cells and make them weaker and more susceptible to cancer treatments. This hypothesis is still being researched and it's still being determined whether or not the cancerous cells will die off when given too little glucose, or if they will find another way to sustain themselves once that source of fuel is taken away. Specialists studying this process are divided on their hypotheses for this research, but only time and rigorous research will tell.

What has been found is that by reducing the glucose dependency of your system, your energy levels and fat burning in the body are both greatly increased, giving you a greater feeling of vitality while you're working with your doctor to determine the most effective course of treatment. Doing a dietary regimen that improves and safeguards your health while you're working with your doctor on your treatments is a great way to make sure that you're giving your body the best possible chance at getting through treatment with as much strength as possible.

Autoimmune Disorders and Cancer

There is a connection between autoimmune disorders and

cancer and it is something that warrants some attention from both patients and doctors. Autoimmune disorders, as you might be aware, are disorders that make one more susceptible to catching illnesses than one might otherwise be. Our immune systems can handle a lot when they're running properly and they are often doing so much in the background and keeping us feeling so normal that we fail to realize how much of a risk there is around us for illness and disease. People who have autoimmune disorders are often acutely aware of the things that are always around them and are more apt to take precautions to keep themselves from getting sick, as their immune system isn't keeping them as protected.

When someone with an autoimmune disorder gets cancer, which is not uncommon, it's possible for their situation to be compounded with yet another disease intruding on matters. Having additional diseases, infections, or illnesses on top of the cancer could mean that treatment becomes a little bit more complicated. If you have an autoimmune disorder, or if you're concerned that it's a possibility, speak with your doctor about testing for those. An ounce of prevention is worth a pound of cure, especially when it comes to compounding illnesses on top of an already compromised immune system.

An autoimmune disorder, to be more specific, is a disorder that causes the body's immune system to attack healthy cells, thus further breaking down the body's defenses against illnesses and causing difficult responses to healthy cells within the body. This type of disorder can start with a focus on one part of the body or in one organ inside of the body, meaning the immune system is focused on the healthy cells in that region of the body.

Certain autoimmune disorders might sound more common to you than others and it might surprise you to learn that some of these disorders fall into the autoimmune category if you're not familiar with them:

Chronic Inflammatory Demyelinating Polyneuropathy is similar to Guillain-Barre Syndrome, but the symptoms are longer-lasting and, in some cases, more severe. In some severe cases of CIDP, the patient is confined to a wheelchair if the illness is not spotted and treated quickly enough.

Graves' disease attacks the thyroid and can cause an overproduction of the thyroid hormone into the blood. There are a lot of symptoms that can come with this like bulging eyes, significant weight loss, nervousness, increased heart rate, irritability, brittle hair, and weakness.

Guillain-Barre Syndrome attacks the muscles. Typically this is in the legs, but it can also be in parts of the upper body as well. This can cause weakness in the muscles and it can sometimes be such a severe weakness that getting around is very difficult.

Hashimoto's Thyroiditis attacks the thyroid and can nearly halt the production of the thyroid hormone and can cause the person to develop hypothyroidism over months or years. This can cause weight gain, depression, fatigue, constipation, sensitivity to cold, and dry skin.

Inflammatory Bowel Disease attacks the lining of the intestines, which can cause a large number of digestive issues like bleeding, sudden and urgent bowel movements, pain in the abdomen, affected appetite, weight loss, and even bleeding in the rectum.

Lupus is a more general autoimmune disorder that can attack much more central parts of the body like the blood cells, the joints, the kidneys, and the lungs. These are all fairly commonly affected when someone has lupus.

Multiple Sclerosis attacks the nerves in your body. Because the nerves control so much of the body, there are a large number of things that can be affected adversely by multiple sclerosis. Treatment for this illness is typically done with immune suppressant medication.

Myasthenia Gravis causes binding in the nerves that makes them unable to properly stimulate your muscles. This can cause a lot of muscle weakness.

Psoriasis attacks the blood cells in the skin and it overstimulates the production of skin cells, creating rough patches of plaque. It can cause itching, severe dryness, and the skin is prone to flaking or tearing.

Rheumatoid Arthritis causes the body to make antibodies that fight against the linings of your joints, causing the cells in the immune system to attack and attempt to break down those linings, causing a great deal of joint pain and damage. There are treatments for this illness, but it can be quite painful.

Type 1 Diabetes Mellitus is targeted at the pancreas and the cells in it that produce insulin for your body. Because of this, your pancreas isn't able to produce all the insulin your body needs, causing you to need a supplemental insulin injection.

Vasculitis attacks the blood vessels and can harm your blood flow and cause other issues in nearly any part of the body, as the blood vessels are all throughout it.

Glucose Ketone Index

The Glucose Ketone Index is the ratio of blood glucose to the ketones in your body. By calculating your Glucose Ketone Index, you can tell how well you're doing at keeping yourself in ketosis and you can track your metabolic health as well.

There are monitors you can buy that look just like any other blood glucose monitor that might be used by someone with diabetes. These monitors will tell you what your numbers are, and you can decide how to change your diet from there.

By knowing how your blood glucose and ketones balance out throughout the day, you can be absolutely sure that you're keeping your body in ketosis and that you're on track to get the absolute most out of your keto regimen and experience.

More and more doctors are finding that keto is a great tool for helping their patients to get past certain obesity-related illnesses. In using keto to help their patients to lose weight and subsequently to lose symptoms, more and more of those doctors have had an interest in tracking the Glucose Ketone Index to make sure their patients are on the right track and doing everything possible to take their health and vitality seriously.

CHAPTER 2: THE KETO-CANCER RELATIONSHIP

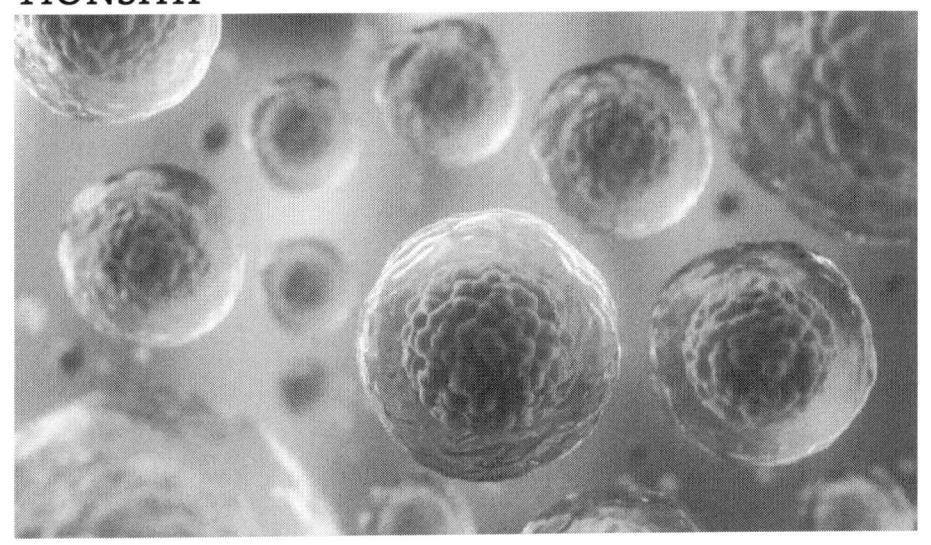

Glucose and Cancer Cell Proliferation

There is a good deal of research and evidence to support that an increased or high presence of glucose in the body can aid in cancer cell proliferation for certain types of cancer. Endometriosis, in particular, has been found to have this connection with glucose.

Doctors have recommended that cutting down on sugar intake while going through treatment for endometriosis (there is not currently a cure for endometriosis) could help to keep things under control. In addition to helping the proliferation of those cancerous cells, glucose has also been found to help cancer cells to stick and make their way into more parts of the body.

It is known that diabetes and obesity put someone at a far greater risk for cancer, particularly endometrial cancer that was the focus of this research. By spotting a high rate of aerobic glycolysis, doctors were able to determine that endometrial cancer cells were consuming glucose as their main source of food and fuel. It was in this research that the doctors investigated the effects of various concentrations of glucose on the proliferation of endometrial cancer cells.

The cells that were given a high concentration of glucose did exhibit increased growth and those who were given a much lower concentration showed signs of slowing and seizing.

Research of this type does tend to embolden people who have been rallying for people to see the use in a healthy lifestyle that revolves around a low sugar intake and a steady flow of high-quality and very nourishing foods for your body.

With keto, you are taking away your body's use of glucose as a fuel source, which is where the hypothesis is derived that keto could have an effect on the cancer cells in a body. There isn't currently a wealth of evidence to support this theory, but there are those who have experienced a much smoother transition from diagnosis through to a cured state. This is, of course, in addition to the medical treatments that are prescribed and administered only by specialists and medical professionals who are very experienced in what they're doing.

Talking with your doctor about the connection between glucose as a cancer cell food and ketosis could be a great first step in aiding your healing process as much as you possibly can.

Glucose and Glutamine as Cancer Cell Food

We've discussed in this chapter how glucose has been seen to be a fuel source and a growth enabler for cancer cells. What might be more surprising, however, is the use of glutamine as a source of fuel for cancer cells. Glutamine is an amino acid that is considered nonessential, which means your body can produce that one on its own. Essential amino acids are the ones that you must reliably get from food or outside supplements. They are an *essential* addition to your diet.

Glutamine can be synthesized and taken if your liver is not producing the right amount or if there is some other issue with your own glutamine production. Largely, the liver deals with the metabolism of glutamine and it retains a good deal of it for its own fuel. When we eat foods like meat, seafood, beans, protein supplements, milk, nuts, cabbage, and more, our bodies will produce more glutamine.

As it turns out, there are no dietary changes you can make to affect your glutamine production enough to starve cancer cells of this nonessential amino acid. If your doctor decides that depriving cancer cells of glutamine is the answer to your treatment, they will need to get very creative and probably a little bit off-the-rails.

There isn't currently a treatment that can suppress glutamine production in the body without causing damage to the patient in the process, though research is still being conducted. At this time, the only way in which the glutamine levels can fall in the body is when there is intense trauma or sepsis in the body, which doesn't lead to wellness by any means.

At this time, all we know is that cancer cells can eat glutamine and that there are not currently any means by which we can cut off that fuel source. Speak with your doctor about what they know about cancer cell proliferation and see if they can offer you any guidance on your regimen that might help you to make the best possible choices to avoid worsening the cancer and to promote health and comfort throughout your treatment as much as is possible.

The Problem with the Metabolism of Glucose

The problem, at present, is that the regular, non-ketogenic diet causes the body to metabolize everything as sugar. When your body breaks food down in your digestive system, it's divided up and used in the body in the best way to keep you going. When your body turns food into glucose, it uses that glucose for fuel. When there is excess fuel, your body stores it in the body and leaves it for a time when it's starving and can rely on that to keep it going.

For most of us, that moment of starvation doesn't come. We have gotten to a point in society at which food is much more readily available, so your body has stores of fat on board that it will likely never get the chance to use unless the diet changes.

That is one of the problems with the metabolism of glucose. When it comes to cancer, the problem with glucose is that if it's just sitting there, the cancer cell can now feast on those stores and keep itself going for a long, long time.

Keep in mind the ratios at play. Just a few tiny cells have all those stores of glucose to use. Think of how much growing those tiny cells can do with all of that fuel. This is where it becomes crucial to a) start cancer treatment as quickly as possible b) cut off the steady flow of glucose into the body that isn't being used and c) start to vastly decimate those stores of fat.

Doing all these things at once can give you a much greater chance to starve those cancer cells and to make them much more receptive to the treatments you and your doctor have agreed upon.

For many who are going through cancer treatment, you will experience a loss of appetite that will make it seem much easier to stick to a dietary regimen that doesn't include lots of things that cancer cells can use to thrive. This is a give and take with the fact that the cancer treatments can often be very hard on the body and it can be hard to enjoy the results of your dietary triumphs until later in the game.

Still, doing everything you can to aid your doctor to rid you of those cancer cells as quickly and as easily as possible can be very empowering. In a typically frightening situation in which many people don't see the possibility for control, it can give you the very real sense that you're having an effect on your treatment and that you're influencing the outcome of it with your actions.

Here's too controlling what little we can in this crazy world!

CHAPTER 3: KETOSIS

What is Ketosis?

Ketosis is a metabolic process, which means it's a process that has to do with the way you process food after you eat it. This is the process that kicks into action when your body isn't getting enough glucose from the foods you're eating to allow it to derive fuel from it. When your body doesn't have anything new to work off of in terms of incoming glucose, it turns its attention to the stores of fat that are already in the body. When fuel cannot be used by the body, it's turned into glycogen and stored in the body, creating excess body fat.

Most of us have some measure of fat stored in our body, and some of us have more than others. While having a percentage of body fat is a good thing that keeps you healthy and your body working properly, exceeding those percentages can leave you a little bit exposed when it comes to illnesses. It turns out that more and more illnesses are being discovered to have a connection with overabundant body fat and their proliferation.

When your body is in ketosis, your body is making use of those glycogen stores and helping you to whittle them down little by little each day so you no longer have those excess stores of fat in your body. It might take some time, months in most cases, to get where you want to be, but there's nothing wrong with that. We're all different and we're all taking our health into our own hands. What matters is that you're doing what's right for your health and that you're helping your body to heal from anything that could currently be affecting it, or which could be affecting it in the future.

With ketosis, your body gets into a mode of living on the fat that's in your body. What helps your body to continue working on this process is a measured intake of protein, enough fats to help keep things rolling smoothly, and just enough carbs to help things along without alerting your body that it's time to stop taking away from those stores of fat in your body. Once you've gotten into ketosis, your body will take on a 24-hour cycle of burning fat and flushing it out of the system. This will keep you completely energized and it will also mean that you're losing weight on a more consistent basis with keto than any other dietary regimen that's out there.

How do I Get into Ketosis?

Getting into ketosis is something that happens when you follow the ketogenic diet. It's nearly inevitable if you're following all the percentages and ratios that are right for your body.

There are some very effective ways in which you can make sure that you're getting into ketosis:

1. Drastically reduce your carb consumption per day.

You are going to be taking your carb consumption down to a serving or less per day and it's best to make sure that those carbs come from healthy sources like vegetables and are flanked by lots of dietary fiber.

By making sure that your carb intake is very low, you are taking that extra step to prevent more glycogen stores from being created and you're forcing your digestive system to make a choice about where it will be getting its fuel. It will have no choice but to default to those glycogen stores and to start using that glycogen as fuel!

2. Include coconut oil in your diet.

While this isn't a requirement of the keto diet, it certainly does help things along. MCT (medium-chain triglycerides) are fats that are absorbed very rapidly in the body and taken right to the liver to be converted into ketones. This allows your body to get into and stay in ketosis.

Many people like to stir it into their coffee to add a little bit of creaminess, while others like to make things like salad dressings with it. It's a good idea to introduce MCT oil into your diet a little bit at a time so you avoid digestive pains or troubles.

Starting with just a teaspoon a day is a great way to go, and then you can gradually work your way up to two to three tablespoons each day. As a tip, a serving of salad dressing is two tablespoons, so that works out very nicely!

3. Get active!

Exercising is a great way to break up the stores of glycogen in your body and burn that fat so it's even easier to access and break down. It's really helpful that by burning fat in the body, you can also energize another process which also burns fat in the body. It's one big fat-burning cycle that feeds into itself and keeps you feeling your best.

4. Eat lots of healthy fats.

Enjoy things like salmon, nuts, avocados, and other healthy foods that are high in natural, clean fats. When you do this, you're giving your body all the fuel it needs to continue burning those stores of glycogen in your body!

What Things Could Take Me Out of Ketosis?

Here are some things that can take you out of ketosis:

1. Too much protein.

By taking on too much protein, your body could be thrown off of its purpose for burning the stores of glycogen in the body. Eating too much protein can mean that you're eating too many calories as well, and it can cause difficulty for the system to zero in on the parts of the body that need help the most. Try keeping your protein intake at the right level. Don't eat less than you need in order to get by, but also don't eat more than you need, or you will knock yourself out of ketosis.

2. Artificial sweeteners.

Artificial sweeteners like aspartame, sucralose, and others can knock you out of ketosis. This doesn't include the natural, sugar-free sweeteners like xylitol, allulose, and others that fall into that category.

If you are someone who enjoys a lot of diet products like candies and sodas, you will not find a place for them on this diet, unfortunately. Eating and drinking those sweeteners with regularity will make it impossible for your body to stay in ketosis.

3. Not being active enough.

By being sedentary, you're giving yourself a lot of opportunities for things like snacking and you're keeping your body from contributing to that whole fat-burning cycle. If you find that your body isn't producing enough ketones, but you feel like you're doing everything right, consider ramping up your physical activity and doing a little bit more with your time throughout the day.

4. Too many carbs in your diet.

This is the biggest offender. People will think that because they're eating all healthy vegetables, protein, and fats that they can't possibly throw themselves out of ketosis. However, if you're eating too many vegetables with carbs in them, you can still throw yourself out of ketosis with that intake. Then you end up throwing yourself off your streak of progress without even enjoying a cheat meal!

Is Ketosis Vital to Keto and to Fighting Cancer?

Ketosis is absolutely vital to losing weight with keto. It's true that you can follow most of the guidelines for the keto diet without being in ketosis and still have success. However, it will mean that your body will not be burning fat nearly as aggressively as it could be and it won't be getting into those really stubborn areas of fat in the body that just don't seem to budge no matter what process you're following.

Ketosis is the process by which your body can really jump into high gear, thrive on very few carbs each day, and give you more energy than you previously thought could be possible. If you're eating so few carbs each day, taking on lots of fats, and not putting yourself into ketosis, you might find that things just don't work out right. Something might feel like it's amiss and you could experience a complete stall in your weight loss progress.

If you find that you have come out of ketosis and that you're still eating lots of fats and low carbs, you might not feel like you're operating at your best. You might feel a little bit sluggish, you might have headaches, and you may even have some troubles when it comes to going to the bathroom.

It's a great idea to follow the keto regimen as closely as you can and do your best to keep yourself in ketosis while you do so in order to keep yourself feeling great and processing all the fats that you're putting into your body.

Make sure that you're doing everything you can to keep yourself in ketosis, as it can help you to drastically reduce the glucose that's passing through your system, giving life to those cancerous cells and keeping you saddled with all that extra glycogen.

If you're having trouble staying in ketosis in spite of following everything you should be doing, speak with a professional about what changes you can make to keep your in ketosis for longer so you can get the absolute most out of your regimen.

What is Ketoacidosis and How do I Avoid it?

Ketoacidosis is a complication that typically develops in patients of type 1 diabetes mellitus that is characterized by dangerous levels of ketones and blood sugar in the body. These two things, when combined in your body in too large a measure, can cause your blood to become acidic and this condition can actually be life-threatening.

This condition comes about when your body is producing large amounts of ketones, but is not flushing them out with your urine, as is typical. When this happens, the acidic blood flows to places like your liver and kidneys and can do damage to them. This condition can develop in just a short period of under 24 hours and should be treated by medical professionals if it does develop.

If you suspect that you may have ketoacidosis, look for the following symptoms:

- confusion or feeling like you're lost
- difficulty catching your breath or shortness of breath
- fatigue or extreme tiredness
- pains in the stomach
- vomiting
- nausea
- dehydration
- frequent urination
- feeling very thirsty

If you notice all or many of these symptoms, let your doctor know as quickly as you can and get help for them swiftly. These symptoms can also be your first warning sign that you have untreated diabetes.

It's important to know that ketoacidosis is rare in people who don't have diabetes. If you have diabetes and you would like to start the keto diet, speak with your doctor about the most effective and appropriate preventive measures to take to secure your health.

While ketoacidosis is something that can happen while you're doing the keto diet, it's not something that is terribly common among people who aren't already at risk for the condition. Simply speak with your doctor to make sure everything should go smoothly for you and then go ahead as directed!

CHAPTER 4: A WORD ON FASTING

What is Intermittent Fasting?

Intermittent fasting is a regimen you can understand with virtually any diet that you decide you want to do, including if you're not changing your diet at all! It's a system that allows you to eat during certain times of the day while fasting during other times of the day. By following a structure that you set for yourself, you're able to determine when and what you eat. There are some rules to follow when you're doing intermittent fasting, but there are no dietary restrictions. This makes it perfectly flexible for any other diet.

Dieting often prompts you to mold your metabolism around d a whole new schedule and promises that, once your body gets used to eating at those times, you won't ever feel hungry outside of them. It turns out that that's only the case if you're not loading your system down with so much glucose that it can't process all of it. The theory behind intermittent fasting is that you're giving your body ample time between meals to fully process all the glucose it's produced so that you don't end up with more stores of glycogen in your body.

In most cases, your body will even be able to cut down on the glycogen stores in your body in between meals as well. This is what makes it such a fat-burning powerhouse. Pair that with keto, and what do you think you'll get? Something that can do some pretty amazing things for your body, your excess weight, and your future.

Intermittent fasting is a very fluid system that allows you to make your own eating schedule that fits around whatever other activities are most important to you in life. If you find that you're the kind of person. Who prefers to miss out on lunch, then there is a structure for that. If you're someone who can't stand to eat first thing in the morning and would rather skip breakfast, then there is also a structure for that.

You are more than welcome to make your own structure after reading this chapter if you find that none of the proposed structures here meet your needs. What matters is that you're able to keep up with the structure you pick and that you're feeling well while you're living life on that schedule!

How does Intermittent Fasting Affect Cancer Cells?

Intermittent fasting is something that allows your body to drastically cut down on the fat stores in your body. Along with this, it allows your body to process and eliminate the glucose it's bringing in without allowing it to sit unprocessed. These two facts are very helpful in your fight against cancer, as there isn't any extra glucose lying around to give those cancer cells extra food.

Speaking with your doctor about how intermittent fasting, when paired with keto, could help you in your fight against cancer is the best way to go, as they can tell you just what to expect with your treatments, just how much of an impact to expect it to have, and they can keep you apprised along the way of the things that are developing over time, as you're going through your treatment.

It's possible that there are other ways in which intermittent fasting could affect and improve your battle with cancer. The best way to find out is through researching for yourself, speaking with your doctor, and trying it for yourself under their advice. When it comes to your health, you can't be too careful and when it comes to listening to your doctor, that's the best possible way to go.

When you're going through your cancer treatments, your doctor may advise that you don't cut back on eating at all. You can speak with your doctor about whether or not it would work for you to simply eat at different times to allow your body to process everything in due time. Talk with your doctor to find a mode that works best for you, your schedule, your treatment, and your health. If your doctor says that intermittent fasting simply won't work with your treatment, then you still have keto as a very viable and helpful option!

Don't lose heart if some of the best-looking options don't seem to be available to you at this point in time. Stick to what your doctor is telling you, do your best to work within the guidelines of your treatment, and keep your chin up. You're already doing amazingly at this point by doing your research and finding options that you think might work for you. That shows strength and resolve, which will help you through the worst of what's ahead of you. You've got this.

The Benefits of Intermittent Fasting

One of the biggest benefits of intermittent fasting is that it allows you to cut back on the calories you're taking in, and to allow more of the important things to take the center stage while you're doing a fast.

In the times of the caveman, humans were hunters and gatherers. We would venture out of our caves to find creatures and growths that we could eat from the land, we would get our fill, and then we would either continue to move along through the lands or we would go back into our caves to stay safe from the creatures that roamed the lands. Back in these days, food was fairly scarce, as people were limited only to the creatures that happened to cross their paths when they went out, or which they tracked down and captured. Once a certain plant or animal wasn't in a certain area anymore, they would either move or they would take to eating something else. As you can imagine, this is far more involved than our modern processes of food procurement. Even with the advent of farming, food became far more abundant.

In those times, our bodies adapted a system of keeping us sustained. Much like a cactus, the foods we ate in one sitting might be a little bit too much for us to use all at once, but we created stores in our bodies. Those stores were perfect for keeping us sustained throughout the coming hours and days during which there was no food, so the glycogen being stored in the body around that time had a very real chance of getting used within the week, if not sooner! For the modern human, however, we are eating far more than we need or can use in one sitting and then we'll do it all over again in just a few hours. That results in stores on top of stores of glycogen with no time in the near future that they will be used, right?

The theory behind intermittent fasting is that you're giving your body the time during which it can put those stores to use and you're taking control of your intake between fasts so that you're not giving your body even more glycogen that it has already stored.

The Types of Fasting

There are a number of ways in which you can structure your intermittent fasts. You don't need to keep yourself to a schedule that doesn't work for you, but you do need to pick one schedule and work with it. Keeping the same schedule for several months at a time gives your body the best possible grounds on which to predict that it will be using new food that has come in or if it will need to break into the stores of glycogen in the body.

When you look at the different types of fasting schedules you can do, you will find that some of them are much more doable right out of the gate than some of the others. There is a lot to know about how to do intermittent fasting, so if you're serious about getting started with it, I suggest you look up all the ways in which you can prepare yourself for intermittent fasting, things to avoid while you're doing it, the types of supplements that are more ideal for someone who would like to fast on that kind of schedule, and the best tips for guaranteed success.

If you can't find a fasting schedule that works for you, don't worry about it! Intermittent fasting isn't something that everyone can do and it's certainly not the most comfortable of lifestyles. You might just need to get your introduction to the concept and come back to it at a later point in your life. There is nothing wrong with coming back to it when you're better prepared or when your life is in a better spot to allow you to do this comfortably.

As with everything else that is in this book, make sure that you have all the information, make sure that you're working with advice from your doctor, and make sure that you're doing the things that are best for you personally. No one else will benefit from your dietary regimen, so you are the only one that matters!

The 12/12 Fast

The 12/12 fast is when there are 12 hours of the day during which you eat nothing and 12 hours of the day during which you eat all your meals. Typically you would center the 12 hours over the time when you're sleeping, and you would fast through one of your meals for the day.

Let's say that you decide to start your fast at 10:00 PM, then eat nothing until 10:00 AM. This means that you would likely skip breakfast, come into the day with a small snack, then eat lunch and dinner as normal. You can structure this in any way that makes you most comfortable, so if you would rather skip dinner and have breakfast, then you are more than welcome to do so. Picking the right fast means choosing something that you're most comfortable with doing.

If you sleep for 8 hours, then you're really only fasting over one meal, a four-hour period. It's wise not to eat for up to two hours before bedtime so your body has plenty of time to digest everything you've eaten before you go to sleep. You can choose whether to factor that two hours into your fast or not.

For the 12 hours that you'll be eating, you can choose meals that are healthy and packed with great nutrients for your body and you can keep an eye on the amount that you're eating. It's important not to use the time between fasts as a time to binge eat. You want to eat nice, normal amounts. You want to make sure that you're not going over your allowance for anything like calories or your other macros.

If you are not sure about how you would structure your meals, play around with it a little bit. Figure out how many calories and macros are taken up by your typical lunch and snacks, then figure out how much your other meal might take up and see how all of that shakes out for you. Make sure you're eating enough of the good stuff, as well! No going to fast food places for your second meal of the day.

The 16/8 Fast

The 16/8 fast is a little bit more intensive than the 12/12 fast, and it dictates that you should fast for about 16 hours and eat for about 8 hours. This would mean that you're fasting for about 8 hours of waking time and making sure that you're getting all your meals in the other 8 hours of the day.

Generally, the meal that people choose to start eating is lunch, as this allows them to get out of the house in the early morning without having to make breakfast. If you prefer, you don't have to bother with cooking dinner, and you can center it perfectly over your sleep schedule. It's a nice, clean fit for a lot of people, but it's not for everyone. You can choose to eat your meals a little more closely together or you can space them out depending on what works for you. The best way is to make sure that you're not eating too close to bedtime and that you're not starving yourself when you should be eating.

If you didn't have to eat in the morning, how much time would you save? How many dishes or blender bottles could you avoid? How many gallons of water could you save on washing those dishes and making that food for yourself in the morning? Is that something that appeals to you?

If you're daydreaming about the extra time you'll have in the morning, then this could be the right option for you. It's a little more intensive than the 12/12, but if you think about it, you're still getting the same number of meals and the only thing you're taking away from yourself is more time during which it's okay to snack.

If you're like me and feel like you could benefit from less time being allowed to snack, then this could be the right option that could allow you to open up your schedule, drop your calories, and get the best possible results.

The 20/4 Fast

The 20/4 fast is the one where the difficulty really starts getting wrenched up. This is the fasting schedule that cuts your day down to one meal that you choose. You get four hours of the day during which you can have a meal, you can have some snacks, and you can get all the nutrition that you will need for the duration of your day.

This is the one that I think a lot of people think of when they hear the term "intermittent fasting," as this is the one where things start to get a little bit more difficult. Imagine, though, if you only had to eat one meal per day. Imagine what you could be doing with the rest of your day. I know that some of my readers are looking at this and thinking, "Imagine being starving all day long!" That's not the intention and you absolutely should not subject yourself to being starving for all but 4 hours of the day.

Putting yourself in a situation in which you're absolutely miserable is just asking for trouble. It's torture that's completely unwarranted, first of all, and it's no way to live. On top of that, being hungry is distracting, it makes people grumpy, and it's a recipe for disaster if everyone's just going to be snippy with one another the whole day long. Nothing would get done and everyone would be very upset.

The best way to do the 20/4 fast is to work up to it. Each of these methods could be seen as a difficulty level and it's perfectly fine to wrench up the difficulty over time. Work your meals around your personal activities and the things that mean the most to you and then drive more and more space between those meals over time. It's a gradual approach that will allow you to eventually go an entire day without eating and without too much flak from your body about it!

5:2 Day Fasting

This is the big one. This is the one that requires you to fast for two full days throughout the week. It is advisable that you don't put these two days side by side in your week, as that can be pretty grueling to get through and it can make those days feel like they're lasting a lifetime. Putting at least one day between those whole-day fasts is advisable, and more than that would be even better.

If you're doing the 5:2 Day fast, you're eating for 5 days of the week in just the same way as you would normally eat. Three squares a day with snacks when it makes sense to have them, then two full days in the middle of the week somewhere that don't involve food at all.

This can be very difficult, but it's something that you should work up to. Simply going cold turkey on food for a day can be a little bit of a shock to your system, to your blood sugar, and you're probably in for a whale of a headache somewhere in there. If you're diabetic, I must advise completely against this approach, as this could put your life in danger and no one wants that for you.

Working your way up to this type of fast is the best way to approach it, as it gives your body a basis to work from. It tells your body what to expect during periods of fasting, and it gives your body an understanding of its protocols for when food is scarce. Too much of anything all at once can be alarming, confusing, and damaging for your body.

CHAPTER 5: THE KETO ESSENTIALS

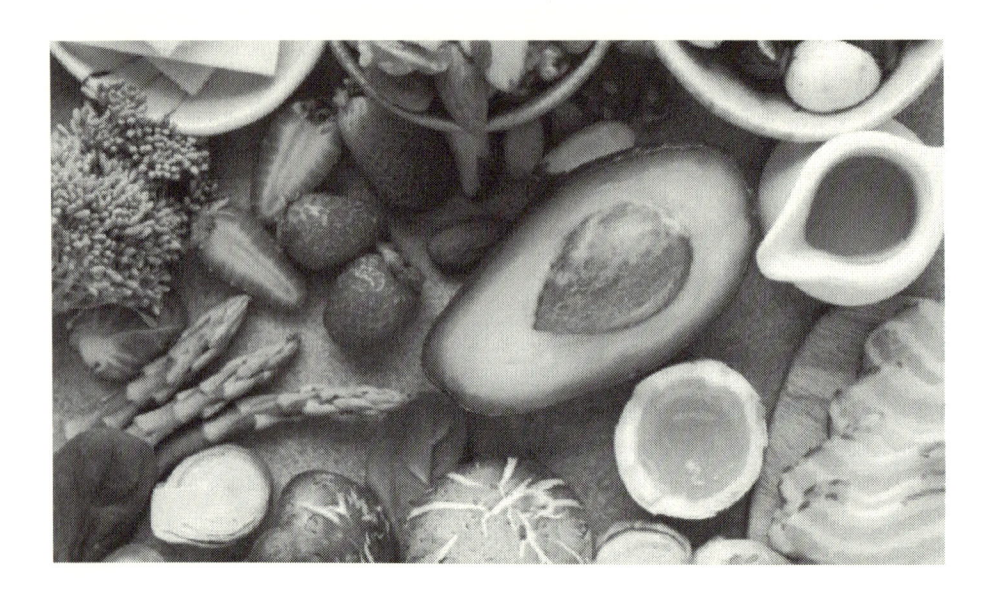

Important Things to Remember

When you're fighting through cancer or any illness, the most important thing to remember is that professional medical advice is the best thing to follow. Make sure that your doctor is completely filled in on the things you're doing at home so they know what to expect when they see you for your routine visits, and so they know what to tell you to look out for while you're doing your best to fight off something serious.

With keto, it's important to remember that the quality of the food that you're eating is always more important than the quantity. It doesn't matter if you're staying with your calories and your macros if you are eating junk food to do it. Those foods are too processed to give your body any real nutrition that it needs, and your body isn't going to be able to make as much or as high-quality fuel out of those foods. Have you ever noticed that you get hungry an hour after junk food? That's why.

When you're fighting off an illness that is as serious as cancer, you want to make sure that you have enough of the right nutrients in your system to fight it off. Unfortunately with cancer, the treatments are so severe that you will often need to eat the right types of foods in order to cope with those as well.

The advice of your doctor is always the best thing for you to follow when you're undergoing treatment for something as severe as cancer even if you are just fighting something like diabetes. Your doctor's advice always outweighs everything else because that information is tailored to you. That information is relevant to your medical history and to your body's behaviors. The books that you read and the articles that you see and the infographics that you find on the internet are only relevant if your doctor says so.

One of the most important things that you have to remember when you're doing keto is to stay hydrated. When you're undergoing treatment for cancer, it's just as important to make sure that your body has enough fluids to keep it moving. If you are used to drinking eight glasses of water per day, eight ounces each, then you need to increase that. 64 ounces of water is the typical recommended amount for the average person. For someone on keto, it's 96 ounces.

I've mentioned this in a couple of other places in this book, but I'm going to put it here again. If you are worried about having to run to the bathroom every 10 minutes because you're drinking 96 ounces of water a day, simply space your water consumption out so that you're not drinking more than 8 ounces in one 15-minute period. Your body can absorb 8 of fluid in 15 minutes, so just make sure that you're not chugging 16 ounces of water in a sitting, and you should be safe from all those frequent trips to the bathroom!

Medical Fitness

What we mean when we say medical fitness is your ability to withstand something given your medical history. Your doctor will be the one to tell you if you are not medically fit to withstand a certain regimen treatment or other undertaking. When your doctor does tell you something like this it is very prudent to listen to what they have to say. As I mentioned in the previous section your doctor knows what is going on with your body and your medical conditions. Your doctor knows what stress will be put on your body by the things that you decide you want to do, and can advise whether or not you're able to do what needs to be done in those situations.

If your doctor happens to tell you that you are not medically fit to undergo this type of diet and that doing the keto regimen isn't something that will help you through your cancer treatment, don't lose heart. You can rest assured that your doctor is being completely honest with you about what they think is the best course of action for you, and that they are working hard to make sure you don't do anything to put yourself further In harm's way.

Cancer can be a touchy subject for people who are going through it and for people who know people who have gone through it. Because there are so many different types of cancer and because the treatment of cancer can be so unpredictable, it can be hard to go through some of those situations. It can be hard not to associate someone else's battle with cancer with one that might be far more complex in the long run. No two patients are exactly the same oh, and we shouldn't treat them like they are exactly the same.

If you have family or friends who are worrying over you fussing about all the things that you're trying to do and giving you constant advice out of nowhere, remember that it's because they're afraid. Remember that that advice is coming to you from a place of concern for you. As long as you have your doctor's go-ahead and you have your doctor's endorsement that you are medically fit enough to go through a certain dietary regimen let your family and friends know that they can rest assured you are doing the best possible things for yourself. That should be enough.

The Right Things to Eat

We've covered a lot about the things that are okay to eat when you're on the keto diet, but it helps to have a section that lists some popular ingredients that you can use when you're putting together your meals for the day or for the week. Let's a take a look at some of the most popular foods to eat while you're on keto:

Albacore
Almonds
Anchovy
Artichoke
Asparagus
Avocados
Beef
Bell peppers
Blackberries
Blueberries
Bok choy
Brazil nuts
Broccoli
Brussels sprouts
Butter
Butternut squash
Cabbage
Cashews
Cauliflower
Celery
Chard
Cheese
Chia seeds
Chicken
Clams
Coconut oil
Coconuts
Coffee
Cottage cheese
Cream
Cream
Cucumber
Eggplant

Eggs
Garlic
Green beans
Herbs
Herring
Hot peppers
Kale
Lamb
Lettuce of all types
Macadamia nuts
Mackerel
Mushrooms
Mussels
Octopus
Olive oil
Olives
Onion
Other lean meats
Oysters
Pecans
Pickles
Pistachios
Plain yogurt
Pollock
Pork
Pumpkin seeds
Radishes
Raspberries
Salmon
Sardines
Sesame seeds
Shirataki noodles
Sour cream

Spaghetti squash
Spinach
Squid
Strawberries
Sunflower seeds
Swordfish
Tea
Tilapia
Tomatoes
Trout
Unsweetened dark chocolate
Walnuts
Zucchini

These are far from the only foods that you're allowed to eat when you're on keto, but this is a wonderful starting list that will allow you to put together a list of the things that you like to have in your kitchen. This will allow you to find the foods that are keto-friendly and which stick out to you as something you would love to use in your daily life.

Consider some of the things that you could make using some of the items in this list and think about how you could make them into a dinner that you and the people closest to you would really enjoy. I'll bet you'll have fun coming up with something and I'm sure your family and friends would love to try a healthy recipe that you've created!

The Wrong Things to Eat

The wrong things to eat when you're doing keto are the ones that are packed with starches, carbohydrates, sugar, processed ingredients, filler, things you can't pronounce, additives that could possibly damage your body or the ketogenic process.

You don't want to eat things that could jeopardize your overall health or your progress with the keto diet. You want to stay away from things that are heavy in carbs, heavy in bad cholesterol, heavy in trans fats, and low on the things that your body needs like vitamins, minerals, electrolytes, and the macros that you should be watching for.

There are a lot of things that have hit the market in the last few years that are miraculously carb-free. Make sure, when you're looking at these products that are marketed as low carb, that they're not packed with artificial sweeteners that could knock you out of ketosis, additives that could jeopardize your weight loss or other hidden ingredients that could insidiously lead you to believe that you are doing everything right only to torpedo your progress.

When you're doing keto the best possible option is to cook at home. Cooking at home makes sure that you know what is going into your food, what's missing from your food, what you need to put in there, and if there's anything that could possibly jeopardize your progress. At least if you cook a cheat meal at home, you know that you're cheating. If you go out and get food that you think is going to keep you on the straight and narrow and it just bombs everything you've been working toward, that is a betrayal. That is something that can be hard to get past. Don't trust the front of the label on the foods that you buy. Always look at the back of the label where they are legally bound to be completely honest with you. Look at the ingredients list, look at the nutritional facts, and look at everything you can possibly see on that label that would tell you if this food is something you should avoid for your own well-being.

Detoxifying Your Kitchen

When you're getting started on keto you want to make sure that there is nothing in your kitchen that you can't have. Everything that's in your kitchen should be something that you're allowed to pick up and eat at the drop of a hat. If there are other people in your house that are not on keto make sure that they are storing their snacks and other contraband away from you. This is, of course, not to say that people who live in the house with you are not allowed to eat different foods than you. This is, however, to say that having Foods you can't eat in the house will make it exponentially harder for you to stick to any regimen that you're trying to do.

If you are the only person who lives in the house, and you're the only person who's doing the grocery shopping, then you need to make sure that there is nothing in the house that you're not allowed to eat. If you have snacks that are stashed away, you know where those snacks are and you will go straight to them the moment the going gets tough. I'm not saying this because I don't believe in you, I'm saying this because I know how the hungry mind works.

We have all been in a situation where we get to the end of the day we've had a hard time, and all we want is some greasy, terrible, horrible, delicious food that we know we shouldn't be having. If you get home at the end of one of those days and your cupboard is stocked with all kinds of snacks, you will eat them, and you will regret it. There is nothing quite like the insult to injury of feeling like you failed your diet, after a hard day like that.

So do yourself a huge favor before you get started on keto, and clear out your kitchen of all the things that you shouldn't be eating. I don't care where it goes, you can give it to a friend, you can donate it to a food bank if it's not opened yet, and you can give it to the kids down the street. There aren't any wrong answers about how to get the food out of your house, just don't eat it.

CHAPTER 6: HOW KETO CHANGES YOUR METABOLISM

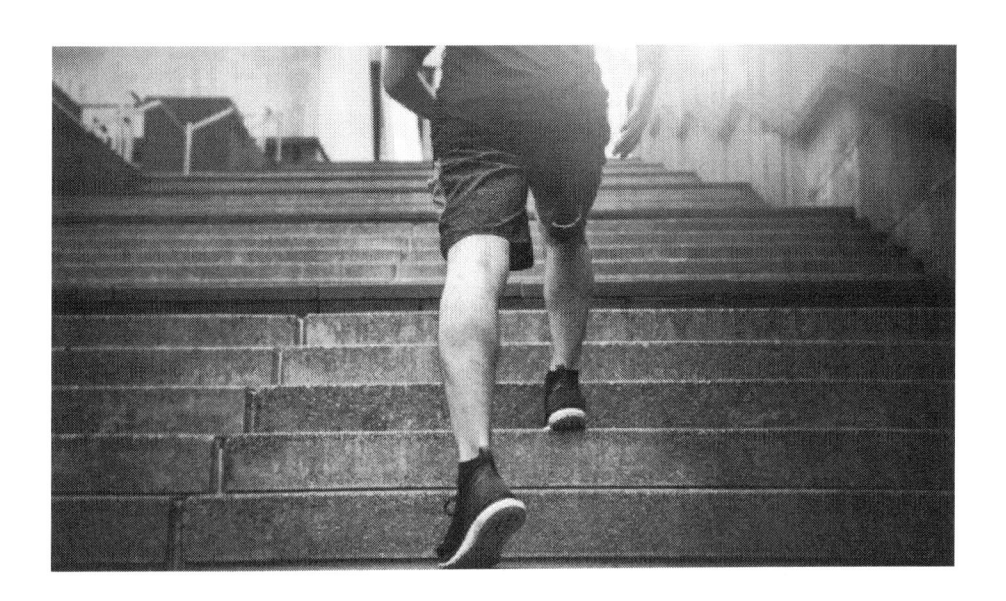

Glucose Dependent Metabolism

A metabolism that is dependent on glucose is a normal one. It is perfectly normal for your system to turn the foods that you eat into glucose, and then use that glucose as fuel. It's that fuel that allows your body to carry on with the essential functions that you need it to do. This is everything from involuntary to voluntary processes. Everything is fueled by glucose.

When you're on keto your metabolism is no longer dependent on glucose. The whole goal is to get your system to become dependent on fat. Normally, when you eat a meal, the food goes into the stomach and is broken down by the acid in the stomach. From there the food is broken down further into its components and those macronutrients in the food are used to the best of your body's ability to use them. The parts of the food that are used as energy for your body are turned into glucose and distributed throughout the body and used. However, because most of us in the western world are eating way more than we need to be eating in a given sitting, the body is left with more glucose than it can reasonably use before its next meal.

As discussed previously in this book, the glucose that your body can't use is once again converted, only this time it's turned into glycogen. Glycogen is what makes up the fat stores in your body. It's that glycogen that we are hoping to break down when we're switching over to something like keto.

Fat Dependent Metabolism

The fat dependent metabolism is the one that is a result of the ketogenic diet. Your body will no longer have carbohydrates coming into it, which means there will be far less to turn into glucose. Your body has to resort to using the glycogen in your body as fuel; that glycogen is fat. Because your body is now using that glycogen as fuel oh, you'll notice that your body has far more fuel to burn.

When you're doing keto and your body is reliably burning the fat in your body for fuel that process doesn't stop in the middle of the night. Your current metabolic process does stop when you go to sleep, which is what makes it a bad idea to eat just before bed. Your body doesn't need fuel to sleep. Your body uses sleep to recuperate and to recover. However, when your body switches over to using fat as its fuel, it gets on a roll. It starts a circuitous and continuous process that does not stop while you sleep. This is part of what can make it difficult to fall asleep when you're doing keto, but it is something you can get used to before too long.

What are Macronutrients?

Macronutrients are the nutrients that your body needs in order to survive. When people talk about macronutrients, they are generally talking about three specific ones. They're talking about carbohydrates, fat, and protein. These are the three that we are talking about when we tell you to monitor your macronutrients while you're on keto. These three things need to be in the right balance, which we will cover in the next section.

When you're doing keto your macronutrients need to be in the right balance, which has figured out using percentages. The percentages are a blanket that can apply to almost everybody, as they are ranges. However, you do want to figure out what the most ideal macros are for someone who is your age and height. Someone who is a 65-year-old woman who's 5- foot 4-inch might not need as much protein in her diet as a 6-foot 3-inch 25-year-old man. This is why it's important to make sure that you have the right macros in mind when you are planning your diet.

The macronutrients are such a focus of the keto diet because when they are balanced in the right measures oh, and when you're getting the right amount of each of them, you will feel your absolute best and your body will do its best work. In a lot of cases, when you feel your body slipping out of ketosis, or when you notice that you're no longer in ketosis by measuring, you will find that it's because in one area or another these macros slipped out of their balance. Monitoring your Macros is the best way to make sure you're on track.

The Right Macro Balance

Keeping your macros in the right balance means making sure that you're having the right amount of protein, carbohydrates, and fat in your day. The way we break this down is by giving you a percentage range for each macronutrient. It's up to you to find out what the ideal levels are for each of those macronutrients and to aim for those every single day.

As we've mentioned, it is exceptionally important to make sure that you are getting exactly the right amount of protein for someone of your age, height, and sex because having more or less than you should be getting could be damaging to your body and to your progress.

Protein: 15% - 30%

Fat: 60% - 75%

Carbohydrates: 5%-10%

There is an abundance of calculators on the internet that can tell you exactly what your macros should be with the input of some very simple information about yourself that isn't very personal. However, for the best possible recommendations on protein, fat, and carb intake for you would likely come from your doctor. Speak with your doctor about your concern about your macros, and see if they can make any recommendations for what you should be doing to keep them in check.

How to Track Macros

Tracking your macronutrients is easier than it's ever been. There are a lot of apps that are available on your smartphone or your tablet, and there are plenty of websites that you can use just as well. The best way to track your macronutrients throughout the day and to make sure that you are getting enough of the right stuff is to log your food. This looks just about the same as calorie-counting, which I understand can be exhausting. However, it's always best to know where you stand.

By putting the specifics of what you're eating into an app that will calculate everything, you stay in control of what you're putting in your body. You stay in control of how much you can eat, and you stay apprised of where you stand. Calorie counting apps will generally have a section that will break down your intake for the day, and show you the ways in which they break down, and what the percentages of your macronutrients are.

With all of this math done for you automatically, it's hard to recommend a paper and pencil food journal. There just isn't any margin for error on something as serious as your health, so why leave it to chance? Get the free app, log your food in it, get a feel for what different amounts of foods look like, get your bearings on how you should be eating while you're doing keto, and then drop the app if you absolutely hate it. It doesn't need to be a permanent measure so long as you can be sure you're doing everything properly.

CHAPTER 7: FAQ

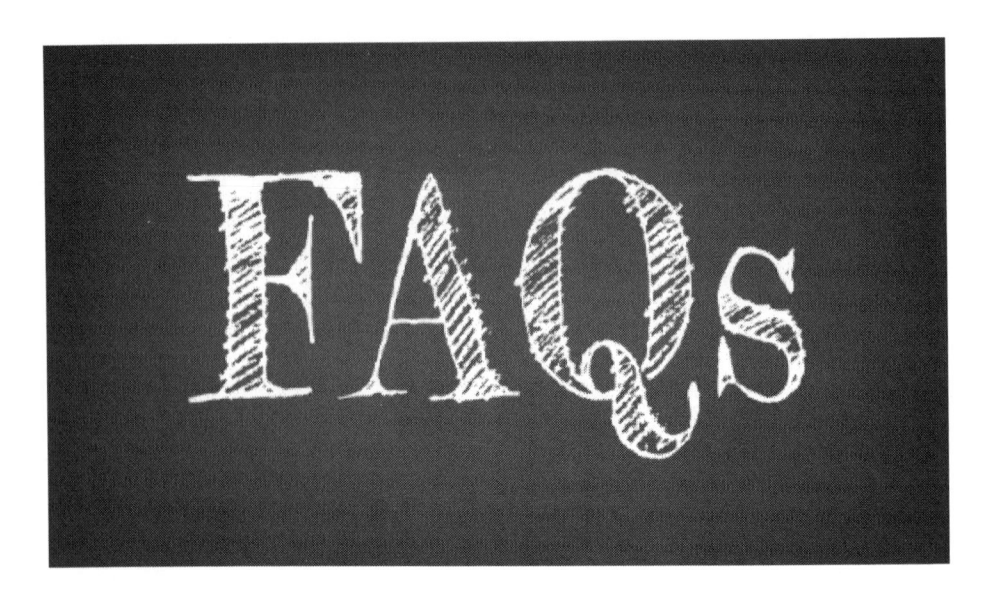

About Cancer
How common is cancer?

Cancer is becoming more common these days. It seems that about ⅓ of people in the world could be diagnosed at some point in their lives. With so many different types of cancer that all range in severity and complexity, being diagnosed with cancer and receiving treatment for it can range from an in-patient visit all the way to an intensive hospital stay or even palliative care. Be aware of the risk factors and be aware of what your doctor recommends to avoid the development of cancer cells in your body.

Who gets cancer?

People who have multiple risk factors are generally the most common people who will get cancer. In the United States, over 1.5 million people are diagnosed every single year and of those diagnoses, many of them are people who are older than the age of 50. Certain types of cancer are more common amongst various regions and ethnic groups, but there is no common number across all cancers and all groups. Different people are susceptible to different diseases in different ways. All we can do is get the best possible treatment and care!

How many people alive today have ever gotten cancer?

In the United States alone, there are more than seventeen million cancer survivors. Some of these people are still in their fight against it, but many others have gone into remission or been cleared of it.

In recent memory, a cancer diagnosis made for a very bleak outlook and it was unlikely for a patient to survive it. Today's rates or survival are far beyond the expectations of any doctors practicing as recently as 20 years ago.

Different types of cancer still have varying survival rates and treatment plan severity, but cancer is largely getting easier to survive with the advancements that have been made.

What causes cancer?

It turns out that there are a number of things that can come together to create cancer in someone. Certain habits and things that people do can cause cancer such as smoking tobacco products. Each of these factors is not a sure thing for causing cancer, but it greatly increases one's risk.

Being exposed to certain chemicals and things that are linked to cancer or which contain carcinogens can also cause cancer in a person. Just like risk factors, they're not a sure thing, but they greatly increase one's probability in developing the illness and some others as well.

Genes that run in your family (also known as a family history) is another thing that can increase your risk of getting cancer. There are many people who have been diagnosed with cancer who have no family history as well, but the genetics are something to be aware of.

Viruses and infections in the body can also develop cancer cells. Make sure that when you get sick or if you've got an injury, you treat it properly with adequate medical care so nothing further develops and causes issues for you down the road.

Are there injuries that can cause cancer?

In a word, no. There might be some other things that happen after a severe injury that can contribute to cancer, but there are no injuries that can cause cancer. You may have heard that blunt force trauma to the testicles or to the breasts can cause cancer in them, but this has been researched and it has been found that this is not the case.

Can stress cause cancer?

While stress itself cannot cause cancer, it can lower your immune responses. This means that you could be at risk for other viruses and illnesses that could, in turn, cause cancer. If you find that you are under considerable stress, try to increase your sleep, get more dietary supplements, and consider what stress-reducing activities you could do to keep yourself healthy in the middle of everything that's going on in your life. If you seem to have trouble with stress and with managing that, consider speaking with a counselor or a professional about it to help you sort some things through.

What are the risk factors?

A risk factor is a very general term that is applied to anything that can put you higher on the list of people who would possibly develop cancer. Things that are risk factors are things like your weight, proximity to dangerous chemicals on a regular basis, smoking habits, genetics, and other things that are similar to this. If you would like to know what your personal risk factors are, you can speak with your doctor and they can help you to determine what habits and conditions put you at risk and how to change them.

What are some of the most common risk factors for cancer?

Some of the most common risk factors for cancer are prolonged exposure to the sun, alcohol abuse, low physical activity paired with a bad diet, tobacco use, exposures in the environment around you, and exposures to infections and autoimmune diseases. If you think that any of these risk factors are present in your life and you think that you might be at increased risk for cancer, then speak with your doctor about how to work against those risks for the best possible outcome for you.

Is cancer contagious?

Cancer is not contagious. You may have heard the phrase, "it spreads like cancer," but this only refers to cancer's ability to grow within one contained host environment—within one person. If you are worried about catching cancer from someone in your immediate environment who has it or who is undergoing treatment for it, you don't need to worry! There are no recorded cases of cancer being a communicable illness from person to person.

Is it possible to avoid cancer?

There are lots of things you can do to avoid developing cancer and you can certainly work to reduce your risk factors for cancer. You can cut out tobacco, you can cut down on alcohol, you can limit your time in the sun to reasonable amounts, and you can improve your diet and exercise so you don't have excess weight as a risk factor. If you would like to reduce your risk for cancer and avoid it as best you can, then speak with your doctor about what your risk factors are and how to drastically reduce them.

Does sugar feed cancer?

There is not a direct link between sugar intake and cancer. There is no scientific evidence that proves definitively that sugar "feeds" cancer cells. There is, however, a link between sugar and obesity and there is a link between obesity and cancer. Cutting sugar out of your diet won't immediately keep you from getting cancer, but it will help you to lose weight, thus significantly lessening one of your more difficult risk factors to overcome! Cutting excess sugar out of your diet as a way of protecting your health is a great idea and one that can keep you from getting illnesses other than cancer as well.

How is cancer treated?

Cancer can be treated in a number of ways. There are four that are the most common and many treatment plans incorporate more than one of these to ensure the cancer is removed and completely eradicated. The four types are: radiation, chemotherapy, surgery, and clinical trials. Radiation therapy and chemotherapy are two of the most aggressive treatment options because they target the cancer and kill the cells. These are the treatments that are done in sessions over time, and which can lead to unpleasant side effects like vomiting and hair loss. The clinical trials are sometimes more effective, depending on the type of cancer, the type of medication being tried, and many other physical factors that vary from patient to patient.

How is treatment decided?

Treatment is decided between you and your doctor. Your doctor will determine the type and placement of the cancer, how aggressive or widespread it is, and then will pass down their recommendations for treatment. From there, it's up to you to decide what options work best for you and for your family. Sometimes a clinically simple surgery and some medication is enough to show the doctor that you're all set and that the cancer has been removed. Sometimes, a more aggressive treatment plan is needed and you'll have to go through some of the less pleasant things that certain treatments can bring, to make your way toward a better, longer life.

What are the side effects of cancer treatment?

This varies vastly between each varying treatment type. Some pills have mild headaches and dry mouth as a side effect, while some other treatment options will cause your hair to fall out. There are many different things being tried in the medical field and there are some medicines that are on the rise as the better alternatives for chemotherapy and radiation. Speak with your doctor about the side effects of any treatment options they choose for you so that you can be prepared for them when they come your way. Being caught unaware of what you're in for can be shocking to you and your family. It's always best to know what the possibilities are.

Is cancer treatment worse than the cancer itself?

Absolutely not. When you're deciding on your treatments for cancer, it's important to go into it knowing exactly how serious the cancer is. This will vary from person to person. It's also important to know that, as cancer grows, the severity of it will also grow. When you're treating cancer, you might be choosing the difference between life and death. Dying of cancer with no treatment is not any more pleasant than going through the side effects of chemotherapy or radiation. Speak with your doctor about the side effects and seek counseling to help you cope with life while you're going through that. It can be traumatic and it can be unpleasant, but life on the other side will always be worth it.

What is remission?

Remission means that the cancer is responding to treatment, when it's under control, or when it has stopped progressing as it previously was. There is a common error that people make, which is assuming that remission means the same thing as being cured, but that isn't the case. Remission is the second step toward winning the battle. (Starting treatment is the first!)

When you go into remission, it means that you're on the right track and that you should be on your way toward a cure. If your doctor has recently told you that your cancer is in remission, you have every reason to celebrate! Just know that you must stay the course as recommended by your doctor and keep going!

Can cancer be cured?

There are many types of cancer that can be cured, but not all of them, and not every time. The prognosis for patients with cancer has greatly improved and the outlook is much better for those who develop cancer. There is still a good deal of risk involved when you're working to treat it and taking your treatment seriously is the best possible way to get through it with no lasting harm done to you or to your body.

When you are diagnosed, you should ask your doctor about the type of cancer that you have, whether or not it can be cured, what your best options for treatment are, what rules they have for you to follow, and do so. If you can comply with your doctor's orders and suggestions all along the way, you will often find that your chances of successful treatment are much better!

What are cancer cells?

Cancer cells are cells in your body that have lost their ability to divide as they would normally do, in a controlled manner. This creates a section of cells that begin to divide at an uncontrolled (and thus unpredictable) rate, spreading and growing. This results in a tumor that can be placed anywhere throughout the body. Cancer cells being shrunken and eliminated is what contributes to someone beating cancer. Cancer cells spreading throughout the body, getting into the bloodstream or vital part of the body that is connected directly to major channels throughout the body is when cancer has become too aggressive to beat.

How does cancer spread?

One single cancer cell will divide and create another. From there, the new cell and the original cell will divide at an uncontrolled and unpredictable rate. This is what grows into something called a tumor. It's also possible for those cells to make it into the lymph system or bloodstream to spread to other areas of the body. Multiple tumors throughout the body are possible if the growth of cancer cells is not treated.

How many people do not survive cancer?

In the United States, more than 600,000 people die from cancer each year. These are varying types of cancer and their battles are all varied in length. Some people have just a few treatments before they're on their way to better health. Some battle for years before they're able to say they're through with it all. Sometimes, even after just a short battle with it, their time comes. Your treatment and condition depends on a lot of various factors. Be sure to speak with your doctor about the things that could be keeping you from the best possible results of your treatment.

How many different types of cancer are there?

There are about 200 different types of cancer that all attack differing parts of the body in different ways. The treatments for these cancers vary depending on their severity, the areas they're attacking, and other possible factors. Make sure that you understand what type of cancer you have before making decisions about your treatment, that your options are geared toward that specific type of cancer. Every bit of accuracy in your treatment makes a difference!

When it comes to cancer treatment and diagnosis, is there a difference between men and women?

Yes, there is! Your doctor will make recommendations for your treatment that are based on whether you're a man or a woman and there are different rates of success for each! Depending on your region, the percentages could be different, but it seems that the types of cancers women are susceptible to are generally very responsive to treatment. While patients of many different types of cancer have experienced a rise in survivability, there is still a difference between the two. In general, this difference should not affect your outlook when it comes to your treatment. Speak with your doctor about the things you will need in order to get through your cancer and follow your treatment plan!

Can exercise keep me from getting cancer?

Exercise can minimize certain risk factors, but it (like most things) doesn't guarantee that you won't get cancer of any kind. Being obese does increase your risk of developing cancer and keeping yourself routinely active throughout the day and by keeping yourself on a general regimen of exercise can minimize your risk.

It's a great idea to exercise for about 30 minutes a few times per week, and to walk a little bit each day. Doing this will help to keep your body in tip-top shape and can minimize your risk not only for cancer, but for a whole host of other illnesses that are prevalent in the world today.

Can a healthy diet reduce my risk of getting cancer?

Just like exercise. A healthy diet can keep you from becoming obese and it can help you to keep your body healthy and your risk factors low. By making sure that you're eating the right balance of protein, carbohydrates, fiber, and fat, you can make sure that your body is getting everything that you need. Keeping your body in the right weight range for your age and height, you can greatly reduce your risks for diseases of many different types as well as cancer. Heart disease, hypertension, diabetes, strokes, and more can be the result of obesity, so it's best to keep yourself eating properly and feeling your best.

Can a healthy diet cure cancer?

No. A healthy diet cannot, on its own, cure cancer. It can go leaps and bounds to help your treatment to act the way it should and it can keep you feeling as best as you can while you're undergoing treatment. While a healthy diet cannot and should not ever be marketed as a cure for cancer, it's a wonderful idea to keep your diet clean and healthy while you're undergoing treatment. Do not underestimate how much harder life can be for you if you're eating foods that don't properly nourish your body and which cause things like stomach aches, heartburn, indigestion, and other difficulties for your body.

Does smoking cause breast cancer?

There is a link between smoking and breast cancer. By smoking, you greatly increase your risk for cancer of many different types, breast cancer included. If you are worried about your susceptibility to breast cancer, then it's a great idea to quit smoking and to discontinue the use of tobacco products. Doing so can also greatly reduce your risk for other things like stroke, heart disease, high blood pressure, emphysema, and more! Smoking even for just a short time can put you at a higher risk for many different things, so if you are considering quitting, you will have a lot of reasons to back you up!

Does drinking alcohol put me at risk?

The key to drinking alcohol is moderation. Drinking too much alcohol can severely weaken your immune system and it can also cause a bunch of other health problems that can lead to serious illnesses if you're not careful. Drinking alcohol in moderation such as on holidays and at special gatherings is not a problem for most healthy adults. A little bit here and there, depending on the type, can be a nice treat and it can help you to fully relax. Drinking in large amounts can cause problems with your heart, liver, brain, and with your cardiovascular system, so it's best to be careful and tread lightly. With a weakened immune system, things could go differently than you want them to.

How often should I get checked?

Going to your doctor once per year for a checkup and for your annual physical is perfectly adequate for your doctors to be able to detect the signs of cancerous growths in your body. If you have a suspicion that you might have cancer, or if you have some symptoms that you think might indicate that there is cancer in your body, then it's best to get in touch with your doctor as soon as you can to make sure that everything is checked out properly, that things are working the way they should, and that there are no treatments that you should be doing in the immediate term to keep yourself healthy.

How does stress affect my likelihood of getting cancer?

Stress doesn't *cause* cancer, per se, but it can severely weaken your immune system. If this happens, then you are much more susceptible to illnesses and infections that can develop cancerous cells down the road. Keeping your stress levels low can keep you from getting all kinds of illnesses and it can keep your body feeling strong. If you feel like you might have too much stress in your life and that you might be coming down with something as a result of that stress, speak with your doctor about ways to lessen the stress in your life, ways to make sure that you're staying healthy, and ways to keep from developing illnesses that could develop into something more serious.

What are the common side effects of chemotherapy?

The most common side effects of chemotherapy are the ones that people will associate with all cancer treatments. Chemo is one of the most commonly known treatments for cancer and it is widely used, but you might not have to go through chemotherapy and thus may never see these side effects. They are hair loss, nausea, vomiting, anemia, the tendency to bruise or bleed more easily, constipation, pain swallowing, tingling or numbness in the muscles and nerves, urinary changes or issues, changes in skin color, weight fluctuation, foggy thought processes, low sex drive, and difficulty with fertility. These are some of the most common and widely-known side effects of chemotherapy.

Do I have to get chemotherapy?

It is not a sure thing that, if you get cancer, you will need chemotherapy. The prescription of that treatment is up to you and to your doctor, depending on the type of cancer you have, the progression of that cancer, and what it will take to put you steadily on the path to healing and wellness. If your doctor prescribes chemotherapy for you and you are not sure that you would like to go that route, speak with your doctor about what else is available. Talk with your doctor about your concerns for the treatment they have chosen for you and see if there are alternative medications or clinical trials that are just as likely to help you to recover from cancer.

How do I find out if I am eligible for clinical trials?

It's a great idea to speak with your doctor about what clinical trials exist for the type of cancer that you have and to see which ones you might be eligible for. In some cases, your doctor might need to refer you to another specialist or doctor who can refer you or start you on those clinical trials, but may patients find those to be worth their time. It is vital to note that those clinical trials are just that—trials. They, like most other cancer treatments, are not a sure thing and you must do everything you can to aid your treatment as best you can. Getting proper sleep and nutrition and following instructions will go a long way toward helping your medications to do their work effectively.

About Keto

What is the keto diet?

The keto is a low-carb, high-fat, moderate-protein diet. It is not a high-protein diet, which is important to note! The keto diet is one that seeks to change the way your metabolism works, bringing your body into the optimal range of fat burning. The keto diet is one that aims to be a lifestyle instead of a temporary regimen, though it can be implemented into your life on any scale that makes you most comfortable. So long as you're eating lots of the right foods and getting all the best results of your regimen, then you're on the right track!

What does the keto diet do?

The keto diet shifts your body from sustaining itself primarily on carbs to sustaining itself primarily on fat. This gives your body the chance to break down and make use of the stores of fat that are in your body. You might have noticed that there are some areas in your body that just don't seem to let go of that excess fat. Keto is an ideal regimen to target those areas, break up that fat, and put it to good use, fueling your body. The keto diet aims to make you look and feel better than you have in years! There are processes in the body that happen automatically, like storing fat that we've eaten but cannot use. The keto diet instructs you to eat only what you need to satisfy your hunger so that your body can make use of everything it takes on, plus what's been left behind inside your body.

Is keto a fad?

Absolutely not. While keto is getting a lot more attention than you may have noticed in the past, keto has been around for quite a while. The process of ketosis was discovered and it was realized that this could be used to the advantage of everyone with a little bit of excess weight to lose. Keto has made its rounds on social media recently, so it might seem that it's something that's fairly new and "in" at the moment. Low carb, as you are likely aware, is a very effective approach when it comes to weight loss. Taking on too many carbs or taking on carbs in the amounts that are typical for the general public in today's world, will usually mean packing on excess weight. When you cut down on those carbs and improve the content of the food you're eating, it's a simple equation that results in greater weight loss!

Are there any health benefits to doing a keto regimen?

When it comes to the health benefits, you can reasonably expect the same benefits as you can expect from any regimen that allows your body to lose weight, to take on more of the vital nutrients it needs, and to drink plenty of water. These three things are always a recipe for better health in the body. To say that these health benefits are exclusive to keto would be misleading, but to say that these things come along more easily with keto would certainly be true. In addition to this, people who are doing keto have also said that they just *feel* better! Better sleep, more energy, clearer skin, clearer thought processes and more. While these aren't guaranteed, they are certainly a benefit when they happen to come along.

What foods am I allowed to eat on keto?

At the very beginning of your keto regimen, it's best to keep your intake to low-carb foods that are high in healthy fats and which have a decent amount of protein in them. Eating lots of fresh produce is the best way to go, as you'll get fuller faster, you'll be getting all sorts of vital nutrients, and you can be sure that the fats you'll get from those items are much healthier for you. Make sure you turn to things like nuts, fats derived from produce, and lean meats that have a lot of great nutritional content to offer you. You're allowed to eat anything that offers you good nutritional benefits without taking you outside your acceptable ranges of carbohydrates and protein for the day, and you're allowed to have foods that make your body feel well and thrive.

What things should I stay away from on keto?

Things that you should avoid on keto are mostly foods that have a lot of starch and carbohydrates in them. Sugary foods, foods that are overly processed, certain root vegetables, and things that are deep-fried will typically have content that you want to avoid. You'll want to avoid foods like bread, pasta, crackers, chips, cookies, and other things that might be similar to this. If you're not sure about what foods you're allowed to have, look at the nutritional facts labels or look them up online to see what kind of carb or sugar content they have in them. Those will be the most key things to look at to see whether or not you can have those foods.

How many carbohydrates should I eat each day?

The range of consumed carbohydrates per day should generally be quite low. Most of the macronutrients that you'll monitor in your daily life on keto will be based on percentages of your daily intake, however, you don't want to exceed about 20 grams of carbohydrates per day if at all possible. Exceeding this amount of carbohydrates per day can knock you out of ketosis and into a stage that is less optimal for fat burning and for energy-boosting. Over time, you will notice that you'll be more able to tell when you've gone over your carb limit or when you've gotten close enough to stop taking in carbs for the day.

What is ketosis?

Ketosis is a metabolic process, which means it's something that occurs during the digestion and metabolism of the food you eat. When your body isn't taking on enough carbohydrates that it can turn into glucose to use as fuel, your body shifts over to using fats for fuel instead. This means that when you're eating lots of healthy fats throughout the day, that you're giving your body a different type of fuel to use. One of the neat things about the process of ketosis is that since your body is using fat as fuel, it will find more of that fuel within itself that it can use! This means those stubborn areas of fat that have been tough to get rid of are primed and ready to be burned!

How do I sleep through the night?

Some people on keto have found that, because their body always has a prime source of fuel onboard, their bodies are operating on much less food intake. They've found that because they have so much extra energy, that it's difficult to get to sleep and to stay asleep. Taking melatonin supplements just before bed, drinking chamomile tea, eliminating screen time up to an hour before bedtime, reading books, massage, hot baths, and other relaxing activities can help you to wind down before you climb into bed and can help you to get a much more restful sleep than you might otherwise have. Try those and, if you still can't get to sleep, consider speaking with your doctor about things you can do to make a difference.

How much water is enough?

The daily recommended amount of water for people to drink is 64 ounces per day. For people who are on keto, this is increased a little bit, along with the recommendation for adding electrolytes like salt, potassium, calcium, and magnesium to your diet. When you're on keto, you will want to consume about 96 ounces of water each day. You might be having visions of running to the bathroom every ten minutes right now, but just know that if you wait at least 15 minutes between every eight ounces of water you drink, you won't have to go to the bathroom nearly as often!

Do I need to count calories?

Not if you don't want to! It's entirely up to you whether or not you would like to count the calories you eat each day. Many have found that calorie-counting apps are the easiest way to determine the percentages of the macros they are eating and thus keep those in check. If you are fine with keeping track by memory or effective planning, then more power to you! Counting calories is a great way to make sure that you're not going overboard and compromising your weight loss goals, but it's not a requirement of the keto regimen, so just do whatever is best for you!

What is the keto flu?

The keto flu is a colloquial name for the sluggishness and other symptoms that one can feel when switching over from a diet that has a high concentration of carbohydrates. People who have experienced the keto flu have said they've felt things like an achy body, fatigue or sluggishness, excessive sleeping, headaches, nausea, and even some difficulty in the bathroom. It's not a guaranteed symptom of starting keto and it doesn't last for more than a couple of days. Make sure you look for all the right things to do to fight the keto flu so you can come through the other side feeling even better than you did before the flu hit.

How do you fight the keto flu?

The keto flu is best fought with healthy foods, plenty of water, and plenty of rest. During the keto flu, many people have felt the urge to quit keto and to just resume eating the same things they were eating before they started keto. For many people, they decided to give keto another shot at some point down the road and found that they simply had to go through that keto flu all over again. You can think of it as sort of a withdrawal from carbs that you simply have to muscle through. Make sure you're taking care of yourself, eating the things your body actually needs, getting all the sleep you need, and drinking plenty of fluids. Once you're through it, you'll feel tip-top!

Do I need to take supplements while I'm on keto?

Taking supplements when you're on keto is a great way to make sure that you're not missing out on anything. Taking supplements, in general, is a great idea because you can be sure that no matter what you're eating that day, your body is getting more of the good stuff! The supplements you should make sure you have are electrolytes. While vitamins and minerals are essential for the body, it's actually been shown that those who are doing keto are losing out on electrolytes, which can contribute to dehydration and the host of symptoms that can bring with it. It's always best to make sure you have everything that you need!

Don't I need carbohydrates to survive?

In a word, yes. You do need carbohydrates to survive when your body isn't in ketosis. When you have switched over your metabolic processes and when you have changed your body's fuel source to fat, you need far fewer carbohydrates in your diet to keep you going. If you're worried that won't be doing well without carbohydrates in your diet, consider giving it a 30-day test. Try keto for 30 days with no pressure to continue beyond that point. If you find that you don't like the way you feel, if you can't find the balance and energy with keto that you can while eating carbohydrates, then maybe keto isn't for you. There is no diet that is ideal for everyone, so be confident in doing what is best for you!

Will I feel sluggish or cloudy while doing keto?

There might be a period in the beginning when you feel quite sluggish. This is typically because your body is getting used to how few carbohydrates you're eating and it won't last for very long. Once your body has switched over to using fat as fuel, you'll find that your energy levels far surpass anything you have previously experienced without caffeine or other aids. If you find that your sluggishness doesn't let up in due time, then it could be that keto isn't for you. Make sure you're getting all your nutrients in the right measure, that you're getting plenty of sleep, plenty of water, and that you're taking proper care of yourself!

Are there dangers to being in ketosis?

The biggest thing that could present a problem for someone in ketosis is something called ketoacidosis. Ketoacidosis is a condition that presents itself when there are too many ketones in the body that aren't being flushed out regularly. Symptoms of ketoacidosis are generally extreme thirst, frequent trips to the bathroom, confusion or lack of bearing in your surroundings, fatigue, and a fruity-smelling breath. The ketones your body produces have a fruity scent to them, so you will smell that either in your urine or on your breath. If you smell them in your urine, it means your body is purging them. If you smell them in your breath, it means you might need to speak with a doctor about how to proceed. In many cases when ketoacidosis develops, the first and best answer is to stop doing keto, but doing so with the advice of a doctor is safest.

Some keto dieters have had headaches; why is that?

There are a couple of reasons why someone on keto might get headaches. The first reason is dehydration. Too many people on keto fail to realize just how much their bodies need extra water and extra electrolytes while they're doing keto. You will need about 96 ounces of water every single day, and you will want to make sure that you're taking some kind of electrolyte supplement throughout the day as well. There are sugar-free water enhancers you can get at the grocery store which contain electrolytes and a range of different pleasant flavors you can put in your water. If you're someone who doesn't enjoy plain water, this could be an ideal solution for you!

Another reason keto dieters might have headaches is because they're not eating enough out of fear that they're going to tip their macros. It's a great idea to closely track your intake in the beginning until you can get a feel for the things that you need throughout the day. Get the right amount of protein, plenty of fat, and just the right amount of carbs in your day and you should find that your headaches subside with that proper nutrition.

Inadequate sleep can also lead to headaches, so do many sure that you're getting all the sleep you need! Taking melatonin, stretching before bed, meditating, doing yoga, drinking chamomile tea, coloring, or reading can all be helpful wind-down activities to allow you to get all the sleep you need to avoid headaches.

Do keto dieters ever feel tired and weak as a result of cutting out carbs?

In the very beginning, you might find that this is the case.

It's not uncommon for your body to react negatively to having to cut down on the amount of carbs that it can use for fuel. However, this isn't something that will typically last for a long time. Usually, this feeling will wear off in just a few days and, once your body switches over to using fat for fuel, you will find that any sluggishness is gone and that you have more energy than you did before you started keto.

If you find that the sluggishness isn't wearing off, you might want to consider whether or not keto is the right regimen for you and your nutritional needs. Your doctor can help you to more appropriately evaluate this and it's always important to remember that there is no diet that is perfect for everyone!

Do I have to give up alcohol entirely when doing keto?

No, you don't! With alcohol, the key is moderation. This should be the case on any regimen, keto or otherwise. Alcohol can stall your progress with keto if consumed too frequently, but every once in a while and on special occasions is perfectly fine. It might be a good idea to give yourself a solid foundation for starting your keto regimen, so your body can get used to its new metabolic routine before you take your first drink. Doing so can help you to get used to how much more quickly that alcohol will hit your system. Be sure to take it slow when you drink for that first time, because it might surprise you.

Is it safe to do keto with Type 2 diabetes?

Many people have found keto to be a great help to them in overcoming the symptoms of their type 2 diabetes. The key is to stay in contact with your doctor about what you're doing, how you're feeling, and to make sure that your doctor doesn't have any other recommendations for the things you should be doing to manage your type 2 diabetes.

In many cases, weight loss is enough of a relief on the system to alleviate type 2 diabetes and to facilitate better production and processing of insulin in the body, thus making any injections and blood sugar monitoring a thing of the past. By staying in contact with your doctor while you diet, you can be sure you know when you're done with your type 2 medications and routines.

I see a lot of eggs in the keto recipes that I find online. Don't those have a lot of cholesterol?

Eggs have gotten a bad reputation over the past few decades with the discovery of, and investigation into cholesterol. It turns out that there are good types and bad types. With eggs, you're getting the good kind as well as a good amount of protein and healthy fats. Eggs are a great food source, as they contain all the good stuff your body needs and nothing it doesn't! If you're worried about your cholesterol, speak with your doctor about ways to mitigate your cholesterol intake and be sure to check the labels on foods before eating them. Cholesterol values on the nutritional labels for processed foods are typically the ones you want to look out for, so be watchful!

I'm worried about having too much cholesterol in my diet if I up my fat intake; how can I keep myself healthy?

The best rule to follow when you're worried about adding fat and cholesterol to your diet is to defer to the quality of the fat. For instance, the fat that you get from a nice, big piece of salmon is going to be better than the fat that you can get from pork rinds, right? You know, innately, that the deep-fried food source is not a cleaner source of fat than a piece of salmon. While pork rinds can make an excellent snack for people on keto and an excellent breading for things like shrimp and chicken tenders, they should be something that you eat in moderation. Salmon, however, is packed with fatty acids, delicious and nutritious content, healthy fats, protein, and things that are great for your body.

If you're worried about taking in too much cholesterol, do your research on the foods you're eating to make sure you're getting the best of everything and that you're not stepping out of safe ranges. Speak with your doctor about what your weekly intake looks like and see if they have any recommendations on ways in which you should cut back.

Should I start using artificial sweeteners while I'm doing keto?

If you can avoid it, it's best to stay away from chemical sweeteners as they can actually cause a little bit of damage to the body and to your metabolic processes. Fortunately, however, there are plenty of plant-based sweeteners that have zero sugar and zero calories. Look for things like coconut sugar, monk fruit sugar, stevia, xylitol, erythritol, and several other proprietary blends and types that are on the market under various brands. Make sure you try a few to find the one that suits you best and make use of it for things like your coffee, baking, and anything else that might otherwise call for sugar.

Can cutting out carbs and lowering my protein intake decrease my muscle mass?

There are a lot of factors that can contribute to lowering muscle mass, but it is possible for lowering protein to have that effect. However, if you allow for a short fluctuation period when you first get started, you will find that your energy levels will go back up again and you can do more to build more muscle. The protein you're allowed to take in on keto will be enough to aid your muscles in their recuperation periods and to allow you to build muscle. Just be patient with your body in the first couple of weeks on keto, as it's going through some pretty big changes, and a lot of them all at once. Forcing yourself into the gym for several hours a week will only make life a bit more difficult for you!

Can a low-carb diet really make my urine smell sweeter?

Ketones have a sweet, almost fruity smell to them. When those ketones are expelled through your urine, they can have a tendency to make your urine smell sweet or fruity. This might catch you off-guard the first time it happens, but there really is nothing to worry about if you notice this. Watch for the fruity smell, though. If you notice that the smell is coming from your saliva instead of from your urine, you might want to speak with your doctor about the possibility of having developed ketoacidosis. Earlier in this section, I explained that this is the condition that comes about when the body isn't expelling ketones in the proper measure and your body is dealing with a buildup of ketones. It's important to remedy ketoacidosis as quickly as possible, so don't sleep on it if you think you might have developed it.

I have a sweet tooth; does being on keto mean I can never have sweets of any kind?

Luckily for you, there are *plenty* of keto-friendly dessert recipes out there. Smoothies, shakes, ice creams, cookies, cakes, and so much more. You can make these with the calorie-free, sugar-free sweeteners I mentioned earlier in this section. They satisfy your sweet tooth and they give you some fun projects to do in the kitchen! In addition to this, while you're doing keto and you've gotten completely stable on your regimen, you can make some more allowances for the occasional indulgence in a dessert here or there. It's important to exercise restraint and to have these only in moderation, but between the sugar-free sweets and the occasional bona fide dessert, you should find that your sweet tooth has no power over you here!

What is the best way to fight cravings?

When you first start keto, you might find that you feel the urge to snack on lots of things and you can't keep the thought of all your favorite carby, crunchy, delicious snacks from your mind. Alas, you are human and it is only to be expected when you've cut these things out! However, you can fight against those cravings by filling in with foods that are rich in healthy fats and which provide a satisfying crunch. Consider trying cashews or almonds as a snack, as well as other snacks like beef jerky, fat bombs, and others. Try also eating before you're hungry. By eating before you're hungry, it doesn't give your brain time to fill in the blanks with anything it shouldn't have. When your body starts to get hungry, your brain begins to send signals and to interpret the signals from elsewhere in the body, then it makes suggestions. "How about pizza?" Before your body can make those suggestions, have a delicious cut of almond-crusted salmon with creamy mashed cauliflower and asparagus spears that have been drizzled in garlic butter. Sounds amazing, does it not? Teach your brain to suggest these things instead!

Do I have to eat coconut products if I'm doing keto?

No, you absolutely do not have to eat coconut products while you're on keto. If you have a coconut allergy or if you simply hate the flavor and smell, there are plenty of other things you can use. Many keto dieters have used and swear by MCT oil, which is a type of coconut oil that is ideal for use as a supplement or additive to the things you eat or drink as a way of giving your body more healthy fat. You can forego the MCT oil and, when it comes to cooking, you can use almond flour, olive oil, monk fruit sweetener, and other products that have nothing to do with coconuts, but still serve the same purpose! If you just aren't certain of how using coconut oil will work for you and you're nervous about it, give it a shot and see what you think. If you don't like it, you're under no obligation to keep using it!

Is keto the right diet for everyone?

Absolutely not. There is no such thing as a diet that is right for everyone, as everyone's bodies are different, everyone has different preferences, and everyone has a different idea of what a good regimen consists of. If you think you would like to try keto, but you're not sure how it will work for you, then give it a trial period. 30 days is perfectly adequate for you to get past any of the bumps and rough starts and to experience the beginnings of higher energy levels, clearer thinking, and better food. If after 30 days, you feel like it's just not the regimen for you, discontinue your use of it and find something that suits more of your needs and which yields the right benefits for you.

Do I need to cut down my protein intake?

It is likely that you won't need to *cut* your protein intake, but you will not need to increase it, either. Many people will make the mistake of thinking that keto is a low-carb, high-protein diet. It is, in fact, a low-carb, moderate-protein diet. This means that there is such a thing as taking on too much protein and causing your body to have some issues with maintaining ketosis. If you find that you're getting stuck in your weight loss goals, reevaluate the ratio of protein to fat and make sure that they're in the proper balance.

Do I need electrolyte supplements?

As I have mentioned a few times throughout this book and in this chapter, you absolutely will need to replenish your electrolytes more often than you might be used to. You will want to have an electrolyte solution that is sugarless so your body can properly retain and allocate water the way it's supposed to. Staying completely hydrated will allow you to look better, feel better, sleep better, and it will even help you to energize. You must remember also that coffee and tea, while they're good drinks to have in moderation, do dehydrate you. Make sure that you drink plenty of water around the consumption of these two things to counteract any dehydration they might give you.

Is it true that people on keto fight with constipation?

When you're getting onto keto, it can be easy to get swept up in all the recipes that rely on bacon, cheese, and cream and forget that we need things like roughage to help things move along. If you find yourself eating more meats and fats, you might find that things slow up a little bit. If this is the case, try to add more vegetables and things to your diet that contain fiber. Fiber supplements are great, but if you can work multiple salads into your diet each week, you shouldn't have any problems!

CHAPTER 8: TIPS & TRICKS FOR STICKING TO KETO

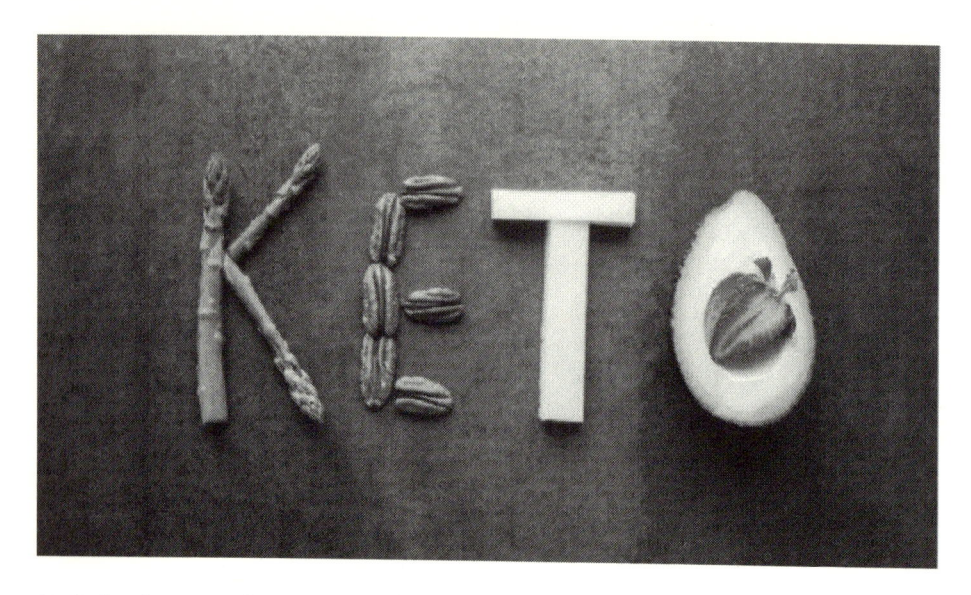

Drink plenty of water. No, more water. No, more!

I know I sound like a broken record, but you need to drink more water than you have probably ever had to drink on any other regimen. If you have always been really good about remembering to drink your 64 ounces per day, you likely won't have too much of an issue with remembering to drink more than that. If you're like me, however, and need to be told to drink water every so often, then this is for you. Set an alarm in your phone about twice an hour to drink eight ounces of water. Whatever you're in the middle of doing, just take a minute and drink some water. If you absolutely must put it off, snooze the alarm. Don't dismiss it, because you'll forget! I know this, but I forget.

If you're worried about running to the bathroom every 30 seconds as a result of drinking so much water, consider this: your body can absorb about eight ounces of water every 15 minutes. If you stick to drinking those eight ounces once every 30 minutes, you shouldn't notice too many more bathroom trips than usual!

Find recipes you love and crave.

Having recipes on hand for foods that you genuinely love can make a regimen so much more viable. Those of us who are very well disciplined can keep ourselves on the straight and narrow for a while, eating only the foods that we know will do the most good for our bodies. However, when it comes to longevity, there's really only so much we can take of meals that we don't care for very much. If we're really slick about our planning and our searching for recipes with flavors we truly enjoy, then we can have meals that make us feel amazing, that don't violate the regimen we've set for ourselves, and that we truly enjoy. Over time, you'll find some really amazing recipes and you'll find that you will prefer to make some pork rind-crusted jalapeno popper chicken at home rather than going out for greasy chicken nuggets that you'll regret less than an hour after eating them!

Don't overload yourself with too much all at once.

This is a lot to take in and it's a lot to add to your regimen all at once. Consider pulling together some recipes and some facts that give you stability and relying solely on those in the beginning. Make sure you have a solid foundation that is simple enough to grasp at one time, then add more as you go along, getting more comfortable with your regimen. There is nothing wrong with getting down to brass tacks in the very beginning and adding more things that make the diet more livable or exciting as time goes on. Doing so could mean the difference between a rough start and a really smooth one.

Plan a routine.

By having a routine in mind that you can use for your regimen, you're taking control and you're leaving very little to chance. When you have a thorough plan for how you will approach keto, what you can expect, and what things are allowed into your personal environment while you're getting started, you can have a greater degree of control over how the regimen affects you, how you feel about it, and how good of a time you have while sticking to everything that you've set up for yourself. Don't let anyone else's plans get in the way of what you know is better for you!

Get all the temptations out of the house.

Having temptations in the house is just asking for a whole lot of trouble. Even if you don't give in to the temptation that's right in front of you, there is always that added pressure on you not to give in to it. It sucks to have to look at the foods in your cupboard or in your refrigerator that you can't touch. It sucks, even more, to watch the other people in your house eating the things that you wish you could be eating. It's best to donate those foods to your friends, coworkers, or a food bank if they're sealed. Doing so will get them out of your house and they'll undoubtedly make someone else very happy!

Keep your refrigerator stocked with healthy foods and snacks.

Figure out what your favorite keto snacks are and make sure that you have enough of them on hand to keep you going through the week. Having enough of the healthy foods on hand can be the one little thing that keeps you from breaking down and ordering a pizza when you're hungry. Having some celery sticks or your favorite keto foods on hand can really go a long way to keeping you on the right track. Make sure you have everything you need for all your recipes for the week as well. Doing so will keep you from getting all the way to that point in the recipe before throwing your hands in the air. Or, heaven forbid, having to go to the grocery store while you're hungry.

Use more seasonings and herbs than you've ever used before!

Seasonings and herbs are your new best friends because they add tons and tons of flavor to your dishes with only a very negligible addition of calories. Make an investment in things like fresh parsley, cilantro, paprika, basil, oregano, garlic powder, onion powder, salt, pepper, and so much more. There are some really basic and delicious seasonings out there that can completely change the flavor of your dish. Having a chicken breast that's been baked with nothing on it feels like prison food. You take a bite and your diet immediately feels like some kind of punishment. However, make a creamy paprika sauce to smother that chicken breast, add some delicious fresh herbs and serve over broccoli and mushrooms and suddenly, you're eating off the fancy menu without any of the guilt!

Stay under your carbs, meet your protein, and get enough fat to facilitate.

The carbs on your diet are a hard limit. You want to make sure that you're never going over your carbs, no matter what. In fact, it's perfectly okay to come in under that number at the end of the day. For protein, that's a goal. You want to meet that goal as best as you can. Going over isn't ideal, but it's crucial to make sure that your body is getting all the protein it needs to build up muscle, to repair, and to survive. Fat is the great facilitator. When you're eating enough fat, everything else will be easier! Make sure that you're eating plenty of healthy fats to make everything run more smoothly and to give you the fuel you need to do everything you need to do.

[Portion] Size matters!

Some people think that, with keto, it's impossible to overeat. This is completely false and there is no reason to think that portion sizes don't mean anything in keto. It's simple math to figure out if you're eating more calories than you're burning, you will not lose weight. You don't necessarily need to track calories or stay super low, but you want to make sure that you're not eating two meals in one sitting. Eat just enough to get full, maybe a little bit less in the beginning, so your body can adjust to the normal levels of nutrition and so you can get used to more controlled portion sizes.

Don't force yourself to eat.

If you're not feeling hungry, it's okay to wait until you get a little bit closer to that point to start eating. Many of us are overweight because our internal indicator of when we're full (before it hurts) isn't working anymore. Some of us have been so used to the massive portion sizes that are typical from restaurants that we don't even check and we just clear the plate because it's in front of us. Put yourself in the driver's seat with your hunger and start to look for and become sensitive to the signs that you need to eat and that you need to stop eating. These will help you to make sure you're not overfeeding yourself and that you're not going overboard in one direction or the other.

Don't eat out of habit.

Eating out of habit or boredom is something a lot of people do and it's something that can cause a lot of trouble for you if you're not careful. Make sure that when you're eating, you're doing so with purpose. This can go a long way toward helping you to eat less. Make sure that when you're watching TV in the evening or when you're doing things that are relaxing, you're not eating while you do it. This gives you a backdrop that makes it easy to eat way more than is reasonable before you even realize it. Consider other habits that can keep your hands busy while you watch TV or do other activities that you might otherwise snack during.

Eat before you're hungry.

If you start to get signals from your body that it will be time to eat soon, go ahead and do so before hunger really kicks in. Once that hunger kicks in, you'll be subject to all sorts of signals from your brain about the foods that you know you shouldn't be eating. If you have given up sweets or a specific type of cuisine because you can't help but indulge in the carb-dense options they have, you will ultimately begin to think in those directions when hunger really sets in. When your stomach starts to growl, it will be nearly impossible to keep the thoughts of those "naughty" foods out of your mind, which will only cut down on your enjoyment of the other foods that are better for you.

Electrolytes could bypass the keto flu.

If you maintain the right balance of water and electrolytes in the first couple of weeks of your keto regimen, you might find that you're able to bypass the keto flu. Those who have been nearly religious in their water and electrolyte intake have found that a keto flu never crossed their mind and never caused them difficulty at any point. It's not a sure thing that you'll get keto flu, and it's not a sure thing that this will keep you from feeling it, but it is a sure thing that keeping yourself hydrated will make anything that comes your way easier to get through.

Pick recipes at the beginning of the week, then prep.

Planning your meals at the beginning of the week and prepping them ahead of time can be a massive time saver and it can keep the mid-week slump from pushing you out of the regimen that is best for you. I know I've been there, middle of the week, work is exhausting, I'm sick of being on my feet, and I just want to have dinner made for me by someone else. However, since I don't have a kitchen staff, ordering out is normally where I turn and that will generally take me outside my calorie and money budgets for the week. By having something made on hand that I can heat and eat will inevitably keep me from making those worse decisions.

Form a support group.

Having support for the things you're going through is always best. If you're the only person you know that's on a diet and you have to go through all the worst parts of it on your own, you're bound to feel isolated and like you have no one backing you up in your efforts. Make it a point to talk to your friends about the things you're doing and the reasons you're doing them so they can cheer you on and help you to make the right decisions for your health and for your goals. You will be utterly shocked at what a difference it makes to have support from your family, friends, and the people who mean the most to you.

Consider adding coconut oil to your diet for more, clean fat.

While it's not required, coconut oil is a wonderful source of healthy fats. MCT oil in your daily regimen is another wonderful way to make sure you have enough fats to operate on. This will keep you feeling healthy, will keep you feeling energized and ready for the day, and will keep some of those nasty cravings away when you're going through your day. If you don't like coconuts or if you're allergic, you can consider other natural oils that are edible to fill in the blanks. Just make sure you're getting lots of healthy fats from somewhere!

Stay active!

Keeping yourself active and staying on top of your physical activity can do wonders for your energy level, your mental clarity, your weight loss progress, and your metabolism. Even just walking for about 30 minutes per day is a wonderful way to keep your blood pumping, your body moving, and yourself feeling great. If you're up to doing more than that or if you are used to a more physically rigorous routine, then, by all means, do what you're comfortable doing. Keeping active is almost always a great decision, so find some activities that you enjoy doing to get moving and work them into your routine as regularly as you can.

Eat more healthy fats.

People who are on keto generally love the fact that it's a diet that allows bacon, cheese, and cream. These are some of the more indulgent foodstuffs that we can find and many diets will curse them because of their high fat (and sometimes salt) content. The truth is, while you can certainly eat these things on the keto diet and while having fat and salt in your diet is perfectly healthy in some measure, it's very important to make sure that these things are not the *only* sources of fat in your diet. You should make sure that your diet contains a healthy balance of good fats and more indulgent or processed fats. Bacon, for instance, is a cured meat. That means that it's a piece of pork belly that has been smoked and salted and brined in a very specific way to give it that smoky flavor we all know and love. That does change the way that meat interacts with our systems; it's somewhat less clean. It's a great idea to look at the quality of fat you're eating each day and making sure that you have a good balance of the best fats over the ones that are not as clean.

Find your favorite foods that are rich in healthy fat and stock up.

You might find a specific brand of nuts that are seasoned in just the right way for your preferences, some pork rinds that you love, some fat bombs you can't live without, or other high-fat snacks that fit the bill perfectly. Make sure you have enough of those snacks on hand for you to eat when you start to get hungry. Having those to hand can make a world of difference when you're trying your best to stick to a regimen. Never underestimate the effectiveness of accessibility! If there are foods you should not be eating that are easy to grab, inevitably, they will end up getting eaten. If there are healthy snacks to hand, you have a much greater chance of sticking to your regimen.

Try intermittent fasting.

Intermittent fasting is a very helpful tool that can allow you to make changes to your routine, to your regimen, and to your intake. It's important to make sure that you're getting vitamins and minerals while you're doing intermittent fasting, so make sure that you're getting all that your body needs to sustain itself. Picking a time to fast during the day can help to accelerate your weight loss and it can leave you feeling more energized and more in control of the way your body gets through the day. If you haven't already, check chapter 4 of this book for more information on what intermittent fasting is, what its benefits are, and some sample schedules you can set for your fast!

Make sure you're getting enough protein.

While keto is not a high-protein diet, it is still vital to get enough protein in your day to make sure that you can handle everything that comes your way. Protein is a great helper when it comes to building muscles, cells, and tissue that breaks down through everyday wear and tear. Getting too little protein can lead to the loss of muscle mass, sluggishness, and a whole host of other unpleasant symptoms. When you set the goal for your protein each day, you want to do your best to meet that number. Coming in under can cause problems for you and coming in over it can stall your progress on keto. Balance!

Test your ketone levels to make sure you're on the right track.

There are test strips you can buy which allow you to test the amount of ketones in your body. The easiest way to make sure of your ketone levels is to urinate on a strip, which will then tell you how many ketones your body is flushing out. There are lots of sources for where to get these strips online and there are a bunch of different ways the strips can measure, so be sure to pay close attention to the instructions that come with the testing kit you buy. When you're able to track how many ketones are in your urine, you will be able to tell how close you are to being in ketosis and if you need to make any changes to your routine or intake.

Get plenty of sleep.

Getting plenty of sleep can help your body to recover from all the work it needs to do throughout the day to change everything over to this new basis of operations. If you're able to get about eight hours per night, that's ideal. If you're unable to get eight straight hours, consider adding some naps here or there throughout the week to allow your body to rest and catch up. Getting the right amount of rest can help your body to digest things properly, to process stress and new information more effectively, and it can even have a profound effect on your mental state.

Cut down on your stress levels.

Having high stress can cause a large number of problems. It can mess with your metabolism, your appetite, your ability to cope with change, and so much more that can make keto that much harder to do. If you're not sure of how you can change your stress level, take a look at some stress-relieving activities that you can do and see if any of them stick out to you. People have found that using things like aromatherapy, journaling, walking, meditation, hot baths, talking with a friend, snuggling with a pet, and a bunch of other things can significantly lower the level of stress that they feel. If you find that any of these things or other suggested actions might help you, give them a shot to see if you can make a regimen of de-stressing for yourself to lighten the load here and there. Life is hard, so you gotta do what you gotta do to keep on going!

Add a little extra salt.

Adding a little bit more salt to your food can help you when you're on keto, as that's one of the electrolytes that gets flushed from your body while you're going through ketosis. It's a great idea to look for the types of salt that have minerals in them, as you'll be missing out on those as well. Instead of going for table salt or iodized salt, go for things like ancient salt, Himalayan pink salt, or sea salt. Just those little bits of minerals here and there in your food can go a long way, so don't underestimate them. If you're not sure where you can add salt in your regimen, consider using it when cooking instead of iodized salt. Most recipes will call for a little bit of salt and pepper and, by using one of those other types of salt instead of iodized or table salt, you'll be adding a little bit more to your foods that will help you in the long run.

Stay away from diet soda.

Diet soda, for some, can fill in a gap they're not used to having in their lives. Some people will drink soda or pop every single day before taking on a regimen like this and find that there just isn't a place for soda or pop on such a regimen. Alternative sweeteners that tend to be used in making diet sodas can cause problems in the long term like headaches. Aspartame and sucralose are not nourishing for the body and can even stall some of your weight loss progress. If you need to use diet sodas as a way to wean yourself off of the general and constant consumption of it, I understand. Just do your best to work it out of your regimen if at all possible. There is also evidence to support that if you are drinking diet sodas, your appetite will spike a short time after you're finished with it and you will be susceptible to more cravings.

Try to get most of your carbs from veggies.

Vegetables offer carbs that come right along with dietary fiber, which is the best way to get them. That fiber helps your system to clean itself out and to get the most out of the other foods you eat later on. By getting your carbs from vegetables, you can be sure that you're getting the fiber that you need and you can also be sure that you're not getting unhealthy carbs that you don't need in your diet. If you're not sure what kinds of vegetables you can have that have carbs in them, just take a look at the nutritional facts and do the math! Here's a hint: onions have more carbs than you might think!

Keep an eye on and improve your gut health.

Recently, more and more professionals are talking about the vital importance of gut health. This is the health of your stomach, your intestines, your colon, and your whole digestive tract. By making sure you're putting the right things into your body, you can make sure that the healthy bacteria in that part of your body are thriving and doing everything they're supposed to do in order to keep your gut clean and healthy. One of the best things you can do while you're on keto to manage your gut health is to cut down on dairy consumption and to increase your vegetable consumption!

Use a scale to make sure you're measuring your food properly.

Measuring your food is the best way to make sure that you're sticking to the right serving sizes and that you're accurately accounting for the things you're eating. Over time, you can probably start eyeballing the amounts of foods that you should be eating or that should be in a serving, but in the beginning, at least, it's best to make sure you're dealing in just the right amounts so you're getting the best results possible without being made to wonder why you're not losing weight when you're following your diet exactly.

Use exogenous ketones.

Exogenous ketones are a water-soluble supplement that you can take once a day to encourage your body to produce more of its own ketones. It encourages the process of ketosis in your body and can help to keep you on the right track when you're working your hardest to stay in ketosis with the foods that you eat. Having a little extra helping hand can keep you on track, losing weight, and feeling as good as you possibly can. Consider adding this powdered supplement to your day to make your journey through keto go a little more smoothly than it might otherwise.

Read the menu before you go out to a restaurant.

Being human and knowing other humans often means meeting up with your friends or family to go out to eat here or there. When this happens, it's a great idea to take a look at the menu for the restaurant you're going to before you go. By doing this, you can pick the item you would like to eat before you go. If you wait until you're hungry, until you smell all the smells in the restaurant, and until you feel pressure from others to make a bad decision, chances are that you won't end up making the best possible call. If you read the menu before you go, you can choose your meal, you can count up all the calories, and you can probably even see if there's an appetizer that might work for you. This small action can save loads of stress and guilt.

Always look at the labels.

No matter what you're buying, you should always look at the labels. Check out how big the serving size is, check out how much of everything is in every serving, and be real with yourself about how many servings you're typically going to want in a sitting. If the serving size is too small for the amount of carbs and calories in that item, maybe you should switch over to something else for the week. If you're always looking at the labels and checking to make sure of what's in the food you're eating, nothing can sneak up on you and cause you to take any steps backward in your regimen.

Make sure you know exactly what your macros should be when

you're planning your meals.

It's true that you will typically want to stick to a percentage of fat, carbs, and protein and that you'll want them to be in a good ratio with one another. It's also true that there is a recommended amount of those things for each person depending on their size, height, and age. Make sure that you get exactly the right information on what you should be eating so you can plan your meals and you can choose the right foods for you. No one wants to have to gain weight in order to figure out they've got their macros wrong, so it definitely pays to check before you get started.

Use a grocery list when shopping.

Always, always, always have a shopping list when you go to the grocery store and always, always, always stick to the list. Buying things that aren't on the list is a recipe for disaster for your macros, for your wallet, and just in general. Don't buy things you don't need because they happen to look good to you while you're shopping. Make sure you're buying the things that you need and that you're setting yourself up for the best possible start for your week. Having the right things on hand can make all the difference!

Eat before shopping.

It's a rookie mistake to go shopping when you're hungry. You never know what will draw your attention when you're hungry. Usually, though, it's snack foods that have no business being in your cart, right? Make sure that you go shopping right after you've eaten a meal or at least right after you've had a good snack. Being hungry when you're shopping can cause you to get a little too creative about the things that you could possibly make when you get home and you might just regret the things that you come up with!

Check ingredients lists for hidden starches.

You won't believe the things that have starch in them when they have no business having starch in them! Taco seasoning is a big one. There is cornstarch in almost every name brand taco seasoning in order to thicken the fat that comes off the meat to turn it into a sauce. Check the ingredients lists for things like that because it needlessly eats up your carbs when you could be using those for something else way better! If you can't find something with no starch in it, consider turning to the internet for recipes that can teach you how to make your own!

Don't get overwhelmed. Zero in on the important stuff.
It's definitely possible to get overwhelmed by all of the things that people tell you to do or not to do when you're on keto and it can be difficult to remember what things you're supposed to do and what things you're not supposed to do. Focus on the things that you know you need to do and focus on the things that make it easy for you to get the most out of your regimen. It's not worth it to get too bogged down in the things that make it hard to focus on the whole reason you're doing this in the first place!

Use an app to track your intake of macros and calories.
Using an app to track all the macros and calories in the food you're eating is a great way to go because it's low-maintenance, you won't miss anything, and everything is calculated for you when you select the foods and quantities that you're eating. Having all of these calculations in the palm of your hand helps you to understand where you stand, what the possibilities are for the rest of your day, and keeps you on the right track with very minimal effort.

Don't binge eat.
Binge eating will inevitably throw you off course for your goals, no matter what they are. If you feel the urge to binge eat, consider having a reasonably-sized meal, waiting 20 minutes or so, and then allowing yourself to have a small snack after that meal. If you still don't feel like your hunger has been satisfied, then it might be best for you to look into how you can suppress that urge. Look into things you can do to distract yourself from that impulse once you've determined that you're not in need of more food and that you've gotten the vital nutrients your body needs.

Let go of the notion that you can "eat as much as you want," of even the healthiest foods.

Unfortunately, many of us assume that if we're eating the right types of foods, that it doesn't matter how much of it we're eating. This simply isn't true and eating constantly can keep you from knowing when you've had enough and it can cause you to eat so much more than you might think you're really eating. Things like lean cuts of beef and chicken are great for you, but if you decide to eat 16 ounces in a sitting, you're going to gain weight, bar none. That is simply too many calories for the average person and one needs to make sure that their portion sizes make sense for their daily activities, age, size, and height before committing to eating any amount.

Talk with and relate to others who are doing keto.

Talking with other people who are doing keto is a great way to get support. Talking with people who understand everything that you're experiencing saves a lot of effort when you're trying to explain to the people around you how you're feeling as a result of your regimen. Others who are doing keto can also help you to find the best sweeteners, recipes, tips, blogs to follow, and more. Talking with friends who hold the same interests as you and talking with people who follow the same regimens as you can make all the difference in the way you feel about how things are going. Sometimes it really helps to have someone you can text about your misgivings, about your concerns, or about your successes to have them validated, understood, and in some cases reciprocated.

If you're not sure about where to start, consider following a blog on the topic of keto and connecting with one or more of the other followers. People connecting over recipes and tips online is a great way to get more information without having to go out of your way or disrupt your routine to do it. You'll find someone that makes a comment which resonates with you, reply to it, and voila!

Prepare yourself for the possibility of keto flu.

While we've provided that tip about keeping yourself flush with electrolytes in order to avoid the keto flu, there is still the remote possibility that you could go through it. It can really knock the wind out of your sails if you're not prepared for it, so just brace yourself. If you do get the keto flu, the best way to get through it is by drinking as much water as you can, getting plenty of electrolytes, getting plenty of rest, and making sure that you don't push yourself too hard. This means that if you're on a gym regimen when the keto flu hits, you should postpone your trips. Stay at home for a while and get the rest your body needs. Putting your body through a strenuous workout while it's trying to deal with all of those changes and the keto flu could be too much and could thoroughly exhaust you. Since you have a life to live around this, it's not ideal to tucker yourself out so much that you add a couple of days to your flu! If you can stick to your diet while you're going through the keto flu, things will go much more smoothly for you when you're through it, so try your best. However, it is okay to relax on your guidelines a little bit to facilitate you getting better faster.

Adjust your keto regimen if you don't have a gallbladder.

Not having a gallbladder means that your body can't process fat as quickly or as smoothly as it might otherwise do if you don't have a gallbladder or if you have a gallbladder that is underperforming, it's a great idea to cut down the fat in your diet. The gallbladder is the part of the body that allows you to break down and digest fat properly.

Naturally, if you don't have this part of your body, loading it down with a lot of fat, every single day could cause some problems for you. This book is not intended as medical advice of any kind, so you must speak with your doctor to verify what is best for you.

The key is to stick to mostly healthy fats. You can also figure out how little fat you can eat while staying in ketosis. This will allow you to adjust your regimen exactly to what you need.

If your doctor suggests that you don't do keto because you don't have a gallbladder, the best idea is to follow your doctor's instructions and find a low carb diet that works for you. There are all sorts of solutions for weight loss, especially ones that don't incorporate a lot of fat, speak with your doctor about the best possible options for you, and make a decision that makes you feel comfortable. That's what's most important.

Eat at home.

Cooking for yourself at home can eliminate far more calories than you might ever have imagined. Eating out at restaurants opens you up to portion sizes that are far larger than you would ever make for yourself at home, and there are hidden calories everywhere. From the sauces they use to the way they preserve the food, there are carbs and sugar all over the place where you wouldn't expect them.

The occasional meal out is fine, of course, people are going to gather outside the house and join up for a meal that is normal. However, if you have a tendency to eat outside the house multiple times a week, you are likely taking on far more calories than you even realize. It is standard practice for most restaurants to give you two to three times the amount you should be eating in one sitting.

You also won't believe the amount of money you'll save by eating at home instead of going out. If you have to go out to dinner with some friends or family, the best idea is to look at the menu before you go and pick an option that lines up with your goals. When you get to the restaurant and place your order, you can ask for a box before it gets to you. When the box comes to the table with your order, you can simply box up half and eat the other half without feeling like you need to stop yourself halfway through your meal.

Try to make changes gradually.

Too much change all at once could be in shock to your system. Feel like you're falling behind on your diet goals, and you feel like you're having a hard time keeping up with everything you're supposed to do on keto, consider backing things down a little bit.

Give yourself 2 weeks to fully implement all the changes to your diet that you need to make in order to do keto. This might mean cutting down your carbs a little more slowly, or it might mean increasing your fat a little more slowly. The best idea is to cut down your intake to the daily recommended for someone your age and height who is trying to lose weight, then make changes to your carbohydrates and fats from there.

By making these changes gradually, you're giving your body a chance to catch up with everything you're doing. You might find it a lot easier to adjust to keto a little bit at a time, giving your body the chance to bypass the keto flu entirely. If this is the approach that you would like to take, make sure that at the end of 2 weeks, you end up fully on keto.

Slow and steady wins the race!

Keto is a process and you might need to make adjustments in your approach so it fits your needs.

Sometimes people give up on keto, thinking that it might just not be for them. In many cases, it turns out that the person just needed to make some adjustments in order to get comfortable on the regimen.

Everyone's bodies are different, and it's not always going to be possible to just jump right into keto and start seeing results. If you're one of those people there's nothing to worry about all you have to do is make some adjustments that are right for you and move forward accordingly.

Don't let any of the keto purists tell you that there is something wrong with the adjustments that you have to make in order to do keto for yourself. As long as you're staying in ketosis losing weight and feeling better, there is nothing anyone can say that can change the fact that you are doing the best thing for you.

Making adjustments to your diet so that it works for you and for your body is the perfect way to ensure healthy sustained weight loss. Going against the things that your body needs in the interest of following a regimen that doesn't suit you makes no sense, and there's no point in it. Do what works for you, and you will see results.

If you have bad symptoms, consider backing down your carbs slowly rather than all at once.

Some people have tried to start keto only to find that there were headaches and fatigue all over the place with no relief. If you started keto and this is what you got, consider backing down a little bit. This could mean increasing your carbohydrates or your protein, or a good mean backing down on fat a little bit, or it could just mean doing things that are a little closer to your normal routine until you can work your way into a more ketogenic lifestyle.

Figuring out your sweet spot and figuring out what works best for you is probably going to be the most challenging part of the keto lifestyle for you. It's hard to know when you're getting started, what your body is going to need and what is going to make it thrive. All you can do is listen to the signals of your body, follow the guidelines and make adjustments where you feel they're necessary. Listening to your doctor is also something that takes precedence.

If you get "hangry," consider keeping snacks with you.

We've all been there. We've all been sitting behind the wheel of our car in traffic, starving and screaming at the top of our lungs at the person in front of us who couldn't be bothered to use his turn signal. However, if you're one of the people that experience this on a regular basis, it could be a good idea for you to keep something to eat on hand.

Having a snack in your bag can keep you from yelling at a coworker. Keeping yourself fed is a big part of the keto lifestyle, because you need to make sure that your body constantly has all the nutrients that it needs in order to thrive. However, it can be a little bit of a shock, how much food you can actually eat on keto and how much food your body needs to stay sustained. Err on the side of caution and bring a little bit more food than you think you might need in the beginning so you're not caught unaware.

Make sure that you're getting enough to eat at your mealtimes and make sure that the snacks you have on hand are enough to keep you from getting frustrated when you're hungry.

Consider adding mindfulness to your daily routine to keep you in control of your intake and cravings.

Mindfulness is the state of being completely mentally present. This might sound like something simple for some of the readers of this book, but for others, it might sound impossible. People are finding more and more lately, but their general thought process is completely dominated by thoughts of things that are going on and other stages of their life. This makes it almost impossible to completely engage with what you're doing when you're doing it. This means that we're not all there.

Have you ever been having a conversation with somebody only to get swept up in a thought process that has nothing to do with the conversation? At the end of that? You might realize you have no idea what the person in front of you was even saying to you. This is because you're not being mindful.

Mindfulness exercises allow you to route yourself firmly in the present moment and make decisions based on the things that are right in front of you rather than based on things like mental notions and cravings. This is why it's suggested that mindfulness can help you to take control over the things that you're eating, so that things like boredom, eating, stress, eating, or simply eating out of habit, don't get in the way of your goals.

Consider meditation as a means for reducing stress and putting you in control.

Meditation, like mindfulness, is a tool that you can use to put you in the driver's seat. Life is complicated, and it can get pretty messy. However, if you're able to take care of the things that happened, and you're able to mitigate the stress that you feel with meditation, you might find that your impulse to self soothe with things like food and overeating becomes lessened.

Cutting down on stress in your life is something that I have mentioned as a form of keeping yourself from gaining excess weight and allowing your body to properly process the things that you put in it. Meditation is a classic resource for stress relief that has been used across cultures and generations.

Consider doing some guided meditations for just a few minutes every day to put you in control of your mental state and to give you the power over the things in life that cause you stress or that you don't have control of. Doing this for just minutes a day could make a huge difference in the way your diet and your life affect you. Meditation like the keto diet is not for everyone, but it's certainly worth a shot.

Look for substitutions for the foods you can't live without.

If there are some foods that you simply cannot live without or foods that make you cringe when you think about cutting them out of your diet, you're not alone. So many of us get accustomed to using certain foods as a form of comfort, and so many others of us use food as a base for our routine. It only stands to reason that if we are supposed to change something that has been a constant in our lives, it's going to be a little bit difficult.

So think about those foods that you simply can't live without and try to find ketogenic alternatives to them. You'll be amazed at the types of foods that creative keto cooks have put up on the Internet. If there's an indulgent food that you love, chances are there is a recipe online for how to make that food with few enough carbs that you can eat it on this regimen.

Many of these recipes will require a lot of work and a lot of skills in the kitchen. It's a great idea to brush up on your cooking skills when you're getting started with keto as cooking at home will save you so much money and so many calories.

Adding a little bit of lemon juice to your water can do wonders for the flavor and for your body.

There are some people who simply can't get around to drinking water every single day. Try as they might, they can't get around the fact that water tastes basically like nothing. In cases such as these, it can be a great idea to add a little squeeze of lemon juice to your water. This gives an extra flavor and makes it healthier for your digestive tract, but it doesn't add anything to the water that makes it less hydrating or less beneficial for you.

There are some who will also add a little bit of salt to their lemon water, so they're getting more of that electric in their body while they drink. I am not personally a fan of the way this tastes, but if it works for you to get more salt into your diet this way, then more power to you.

Citrus fruits like lemons and limes are a great way to add flavor to your water and to your food without adding extra calories. Lemons and limes are exceedingly flavorful, but have virtually no sugar. My tolerance for tartness or sour flavors, you could even eat a lemon or lime as a snack. They take a while to eat, and they're delicious, not to mention the fact that your kitchen will smell great.

Check your milk for carbs. Seriously.

I know this might sound like a joke, but it's not. There are a lot of additives that have to go into the milk before it can be sold on a mass scale. You will particularly find carbs in skim milk because they add sugar to it to make it taste a little bit more satisfying.

In general, you won't find this to be a problem for you on keto because you want milk with fat in it. Even still, you should check your milk nutritional label for carbs before you buy it. Look for the milk that doesn't have any.

Typically, if you're looking out for your gut health you won't want to drink milk as a matter of general course. Cutting down on your intake of dairy can help to improve your microbiome by leaps and bounds.

However, if you are buying milk for a keto recipe you want to make sure that it doesn't have any hidden sugars or carbs in it that could throw you off later on. One of the things that you'll find when you're shopping for foods that specifically do not have unnecessary carbs in them is that there are carbs everywhere. Places you never expected to find carbs, you will see them on the label.

This is just one more example to show you that you absolutely must check the label before you buy anything while you're on keto.

You might notice an uptick in your libido.

While you're doing keto, you're increasing your energy levels by far more than you might have expected. You'll find that when you wake up in the morning, you're far more able to just get up and go. You'll feel like someone has lit a fire under you and you have so much more energy to do things in your day that you might not have expected.

In addition to this many keto dieters have found that their stamina and libido increased after doing keto for a little while. Having that extra pep in your step and having that extra energy in your body can really help to feel more things that you might have considered auxiliary.

Sex drive is a very healthy thing to have, and if you find that, you often have the energy to have sex on a regular basis, then your energy levels are fairly good. As you notice your energy levels increasing, you might find that the urge also increases over time.

With many regimens as the vitality level increases in the person doing that regimen, other things tend to follow. It's amazing to see how many of our mental processes are tied to our energy levels. In general, you might not think that thinking takes a lot of energy. It's never until you feel that energy flooding back and your energy increasing that you really realize how much of your mental abilities when locked up in those low energy stores.

Cauliflower, like turkey, can be made into pretty much anything else.

Cauliflower is like a blank vegetable, canvas. You can cut it up, chop it up, rice it, mash it or do pretty much anything with it and flavor it any way you want to turn it into a great substitute for the sides that we usually put on our plates that are packed with carbs.

Two of the most popular substitutions done with cauliflower are rice and mashed potatoes. By chopping up cauliflower very finely, so that it resembles the little grains of rice and seasoning it the way you like, can do a lot to fill out the dish.

If your family was like mine, the plate always had a heaping helping of something starchy like rice or potatoes at the dinner table. Filling in with something that has almost no carbs in it at all and which can be flavored anyway, you want is a great way to substitute for that carb.

There are people who have had success with making cauliflower, tots and hash browns. There are even people who have recipes for cauliflower pizza crust! There's no limit to the possibilities when it comes to cauliflower, so stock up.

If you're a sandwich person, consider making some cloud bread!

Cloud bread is a wonderful invention that is made with 3 very simple ingredients. All you need is cream of tartar cream, cheese, and eggs. By whipping the egg whites until they get stiff peaks and mixing in warm cream cheese and egg yolks with cream of tartar, you can make little disks of bread that you can use pretty much anywhere in your daily routine.

They make great sandwiches at any time of day and you can shape the bread any way you like, so it fits your needs. If you like to do breakfast sandwiches, you could make little round pieces of bread to use for that. If you're more of a lunchtime, sandwich person, maybe make them in square shapes instead.

These are the types of recipes I'm talking about looking out for. Really simple low carb substitution for the foods you're used to eating. Before you know it, you'll be completely switched over to a new keto regimen without having to sacrifice anything at all.

CHAPTER 9: KETO BREAKFAST RECIPES

Taco Breakfast Skillet

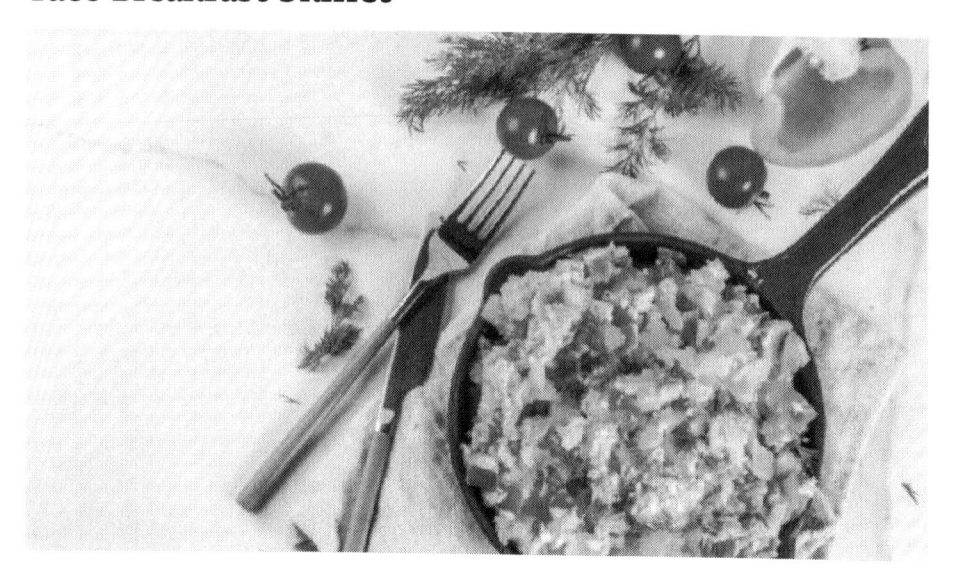

Nutrition
Calories per serving: 563
Carbohydrates: 9 grams
Fat: 44 grams
Fiber: 4 grams
Protein: 32 grams

Ingredients
¼ c. black olives, sliced
¼ c. heavy cream
¼ c. salsa
¼ c. sour cream
⅔ c. water
1 ½ c. cheddar cheese, shredded & divided

1 lb. ground beef
1 med. avocado, cubed
1 med. jalapeño, sliced (optional)
1 Roma tomato, diced
2 med. green onions, sliced
2 tbsp. fresh cilantro, chopped
4 tbsp. taco seasoning
10 lg. eggs, beaten

Directions
1. Preheat the oven to 375 degrees Fahrenheit.
2. In a large skillet over medium-high heat, brown the beef and drain any excess fat to your preference.
3. Add the water and taco seasoning to the skillet with the meat in it and reduce the heat to low. Allow to simmer until the sauce has thickened and can thoroughly coat the meat.
4. Remove half of the meat from the skillet and set aside.
5. In a large mixing bowl, combine the eggs, 1 cup of cheese, and the heavy cream, whisking thoroughly to combine.
6. Pour the egg and cheese mixture into the skillet and stir thoroughly to combine.
7. Bake for about 30 minutes or until the egg mixture is cooked through and fluffy.
8. Top the skillet with remaining ground beef and shredded cheese, tomato, avocado, olives, sour cream, green onion, and salsa.
9. Garnish with cilantro and jalapeño and serve.

Keto Breakfast Sandwich

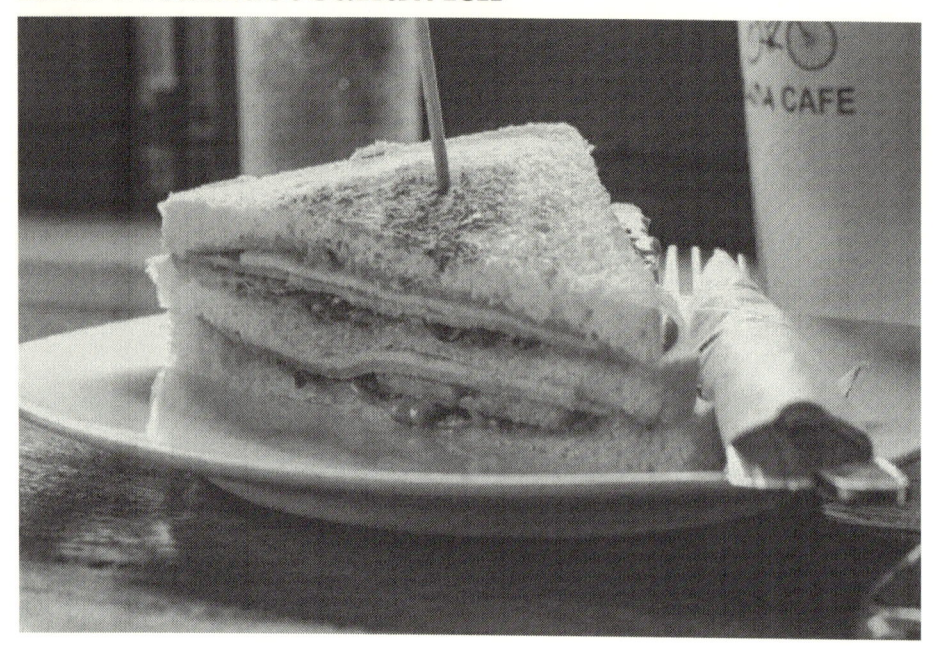

Nutrition
Calories per serving: 603
Carbohydrates: 4 grams
Fat: 54 grams
Fiber: 3 grams
Protein: 22 grams

Ingredients
Sea salt & pepper to taste
2 tablespoons sharp cheddar
2 sausage patties
1 tablespoon cream cheese
1 egg, beaten
¼-1/2 tsp. chili sauce (to taste)
¼ medium avocado, sliced

Directions
1. Over medium heat, warm a skillet and prepare the sausage patties, taking care to observe any cooking instruc-

tions on its packaging.
2. Add the shredded cheddar cheese and the cream cheese to a small bowl, then heat in the microwave for 20-30 seconds to melt. Stir thoroughly to incorporate.
3. Add chili sauce, if desired, to cheese mixture and stir until thoroughly incorporated.
4. Scramble the egg in a small bowl and add desired seasonings and salt and pepper to taste. Cook to make an omelet or a manageable shape to add to the sandwich.
5. Using one sausage patty as the bottom "bun," layer egg, cheese mixture, and avocado in an order that is satisfactory for you, then top with the second patty.
6. Slice if desired and enjoy!

Oatlessmeal

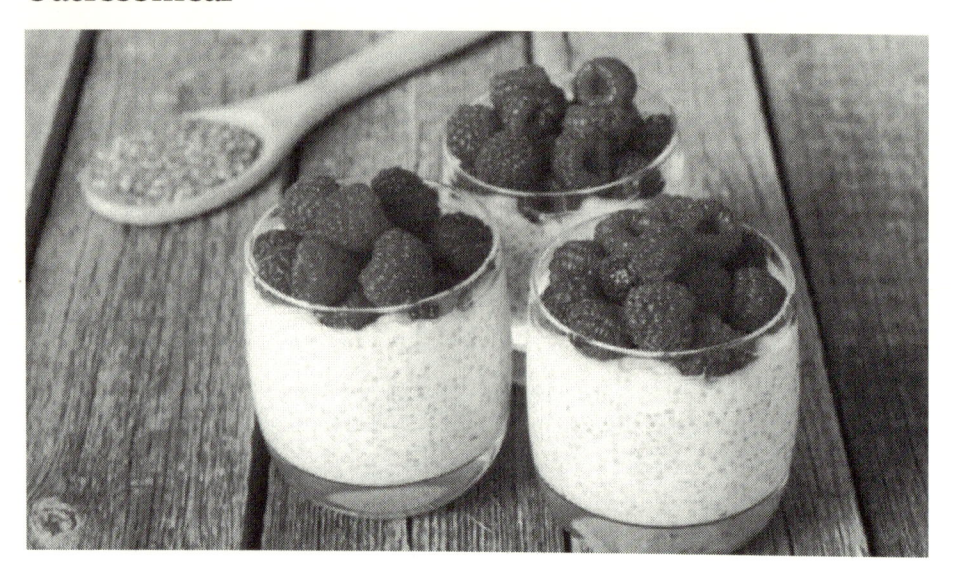

Nutrition
Calories per serving: 150
Carbohydrates: 27 grams
Fat: 2.5 grams
Fiber: 4 grams
Protein: 5 grams

Ingredients
¼ tsp. erythritol or preferred sweetener
½ c. water
½ tsp. vanilla extract
1 tbsp. golden flaxseed meal
1 tbsp. chia seeds
1 pinch salt
2 tbsp. hemp hearts
2 tbsp. shredded coconut, unsweetened
2 tbsp. almond flour

Directions
1. In a small saucepan over low heat, combine all ingredients **except the vanilla** and stir completely.
2. Continue stirring until the mixture is completely

warmed through and then stir the vanilla into it.

3. Top with ingredients of your preference and serve warm!

Pulled Pork Hash

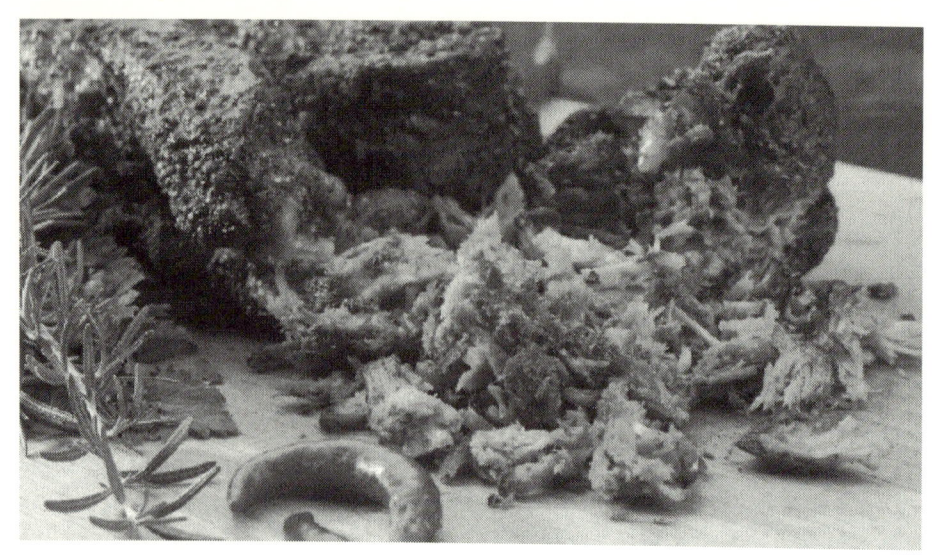

Nutrition
Calories per serving: 291
Carbohydrates: 11 grams
Fat: 21 grams
Fiber: 3 grams
Protein: 16 grams

Ingredients
¼ tsp. salt
¼ tsp. garlic powder
¼ tsp. black pepper
½ tsp. paprika
1 med. turnip, diced
1 c. kale, chopped
2 tbsp. avocado oil
2 tbsp. red onion, diced
2 lg. eggs
3 oz. pulled pork
3 Brussels sprouts, halved

Directions
1. In a large skillet, heat your oil over medium-high heat.

Stir the turnip into the skillet along with all seasonings and allow to heat through for about five minutes, stirring occasionally.
2. Add kale, onion, Brussels sprouts, and kale to the skillet and cook for about three minutes, or until they begin to soften.
3. Stir the pork into the skillet and allow to heat through for another three minutes or so.
4. Using your spoon or spatula, make two wells in the mixture and crack one egg into each.
5. Cover the skillet and allow to cook for three to five minutes, until the eggs have reached your preferred level of doneness.
6. Serve hot!

CHAPTER 10: KETO LUNCH RECIPES

Shredded Beef

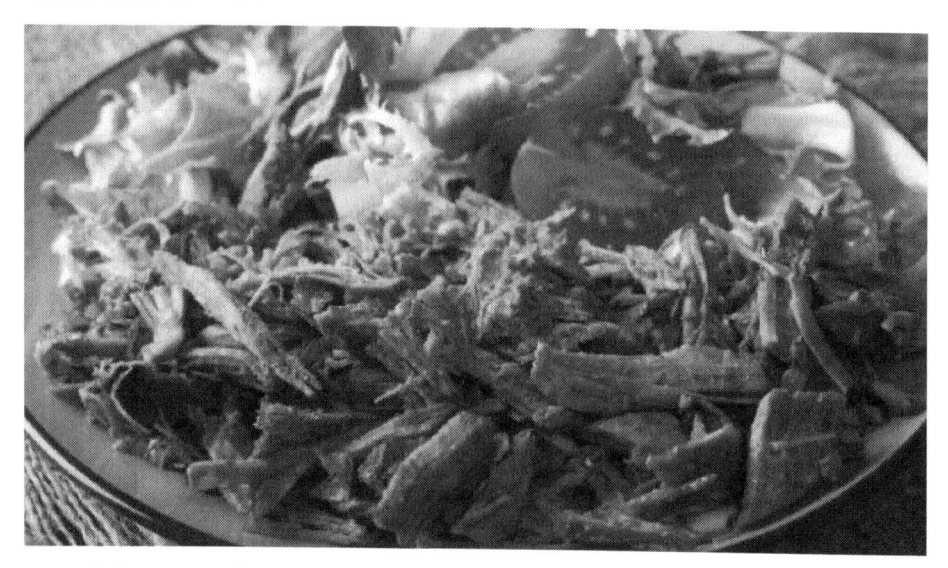

Nutrition
Calories per serving: 656
Carbohydrates: 1.5 grams
Fat: 48.5 grams
Fiber: .5 grams
Protein: 50 grams
Ingredients

½ c. water
½ tsp. black pepper
1 tsp. chipotle powder
½ c. cilantro, chopped
1 tsp. salt
2 tsp. paprika
2 tsp. ground turmeric

2 tsp. ground coriander
2 tsp. ground cumin
3 ½ lbs. beef shank or short ribs
4 cloves garlic, crushed

Directions
1. Combine all dry ingredients in a small bowl and stir completely.
2. In a slow cooker, combine the beef and lightly coat each piece with the dry mixture.
3. Sprinkle the cilantro into the cooker and pour the water into the pot, making sure not to rinse any of the spice off your beef as you do so.
4. Set the slow cooker too low for six to seven hours and turn off the pot when the beef falls apart easily.
5. If you like a thicker sauce, transfer the drippings out of the slow cooker and into a medium saucepan to reduce for ten to fifteen minutes over medium heat, then return the liquid to the cooker.
6. Shred the beef, then serve as desired.

Dairy-Free Butter Chicken

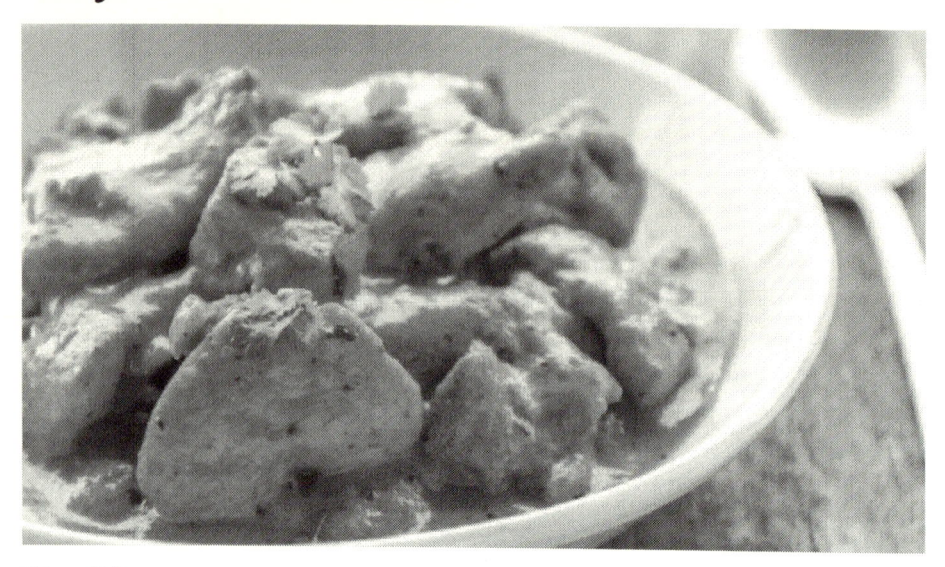

Nutrition

Calories per serving: 304
Carbohydrates: 9 grams
Fat: 18 grams
Fiber: 2 grams
Protein: 28 grams

Ingredients

¼ c. cilantro, chopped
½ tsp. cayenne pepper (optional)
½ tsp. ground black pepper
½ tsp. ground cinnamon
1 cinnamon stick
1 med. yellow onion, chopped
1 tbsp. cumin
1 tbsp. garam masala
1 tsp. chili powder
1 tsp. salt

1" knob of garlic, chopped
2 c. green beans, optional
2 lb. boneless, skinless chicken breast, cubed
2 tbsp. coconut oil
2 tbsp. lemon juice
2 tsp. ground turmeric
5 cloves garlic, minced
15 oz. full-fat coconut milk
15 oz. tomato sauce

Directions

1. In a large pan, cook the onion and garlic until they are fragrant and just barely tender. Add the ginger, garam masala, chili powder, turmeric, cumin, salt, cinnamon, pepper, and cayenne to the pan and stir to combine. Allow to cook for another one to two minutes.
2. Transfer the spice mixture into the slow cooker and top with chicken, tomato sauce, coconut milk, lemon juice, and stir. Top with the cinnamon stick and cover. Allow to cook on high for three hours, or on low for six hours. About 30 minutes from the end of cooking, add green beans.
3. Serve over cauliflower rice.

Salmon Salad

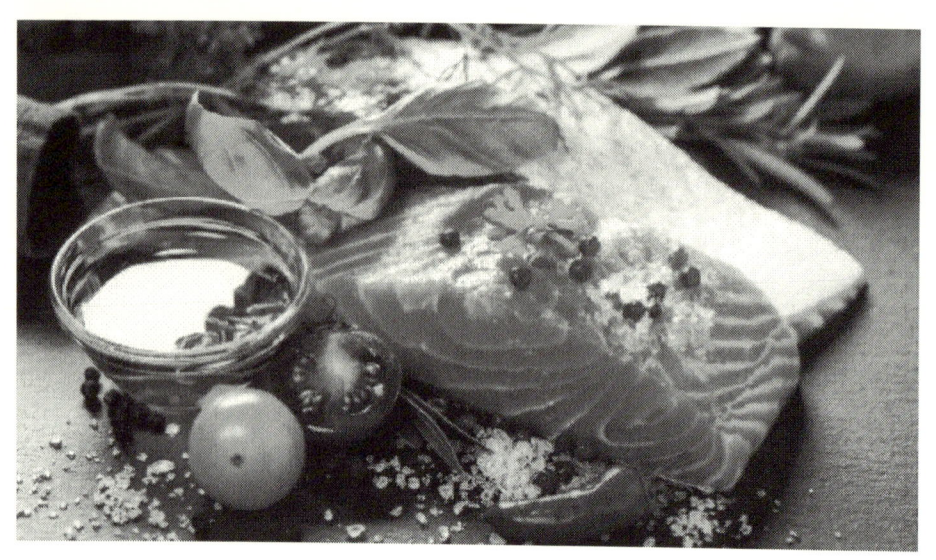

Nutrition
Calories per serving: 575
Carbohydrates: 11 grams
Fat: 49 grams
Fiber: 7 grams
Protein: 25 grams

Ingredients

For the dressing:

¼ c. extra virgin olive oil
½ tsp. Dijon mustard
1 tsp. white wine vinegar
2 tbsp. lemon juice
Salt and pepper to taste

For the salad:

1 med. avocado, sliced
3 oz. arugula
8 oz. smoked salmon fillet, cooked and chopped

Directions
1. In a small bowl, combine all ingredients for the dressing and mix completely with a fork.
2. Combine all ingredients for the salad in a large bowl, then top with dressing.
3. Toss together until the salad is generously coated, then serve chilled.

Chicken Avocado Salad

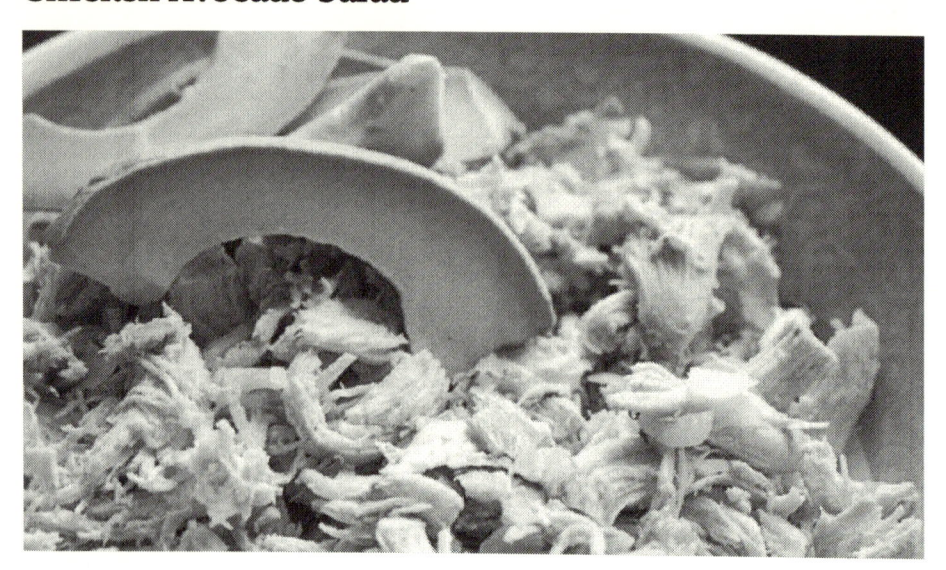

Nutrition
Calories per serving: 545
Carbohydrates: 10 grams
Fat: 38 grams
Fiber: 5 grams
Protein: 40 grams
Ingredients

For the lemon dressing:

3 tbsp. lemon juice
3 tbsp. extra virgin olive oil
Salt and pepper to taste

For the salad:

¼ med. red onion, thinly sliced
½ c. parsley, chopped
1 rotisserie chicken, deboned and shredded
1 lg. English or hothouse cucumber, halved & sliced
2 med. avocados, pitted and diced

5 lg. Roma tomatoes, chopped

Directions
1. In a small bowl, combine all ingredients for the dressing and mix completely with a fork.
2. Combine all ingredients for the salad in a large bowl, then top with dressing.
3. Toss together until the salad is generously coated, then serve chilled.

CHAPTER 11: KETO DINNER RECIPES

White Chicken Chili

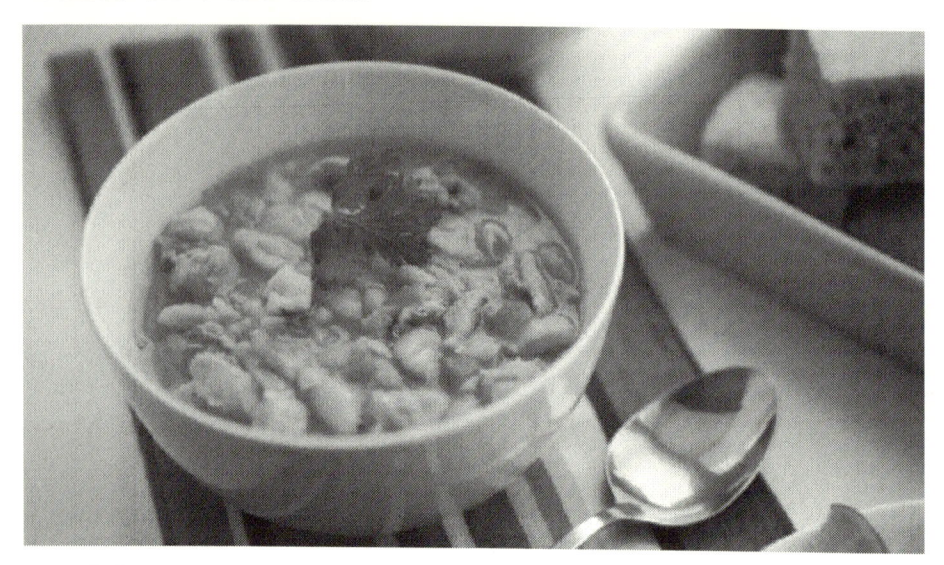

Nutrition
Calories per serving: 591
Carbohydrates: 5 grams
Fat: 50 grams
Fiber: 1 gram
Protein: 40 grams
Ingredients

¾ c. chicken broth

1 ½ c. Monterey jack cheese, shredded

1 ½ tbsp. onion powder

1 ½ tsp. chili powder

1 stick butter, divided

1 tbsp. extra virgin olive oil

1 tsp. hot sauce

2 c. heavy cream
2 lbs. chicken breasts, boneless & skinless
2 tsp. ground cumin
4 oz. cream cheese
8 oz. diced green chiles
Salt and pepper to taste

Directions
1. Over medium-high heat, melt oil and 2 tablespoons of butter.
2. Coat the chicken breasts with chili powder, salt, and pepper. Cook each breast for about five minutes, then flip. Turn one to two times per side until the inside is cooked and has reached a temperature of 165 degrees Fahrenheit.
3. In a large pot, mix the remainder of the butter with the chicken broth, cream cheese, heavy cream, cumin, onion powder, and the hot sauce. Season to taste with salt and pepper and bring the mixture to a simmer. Allow to simmer for about five minutes, or until all the ingredients can be stirred smoothly together.
4. Stir the chicken, cheese, and chiles into the pot and reduce the heat to low. Stir occasionally and allow to cook for about 20 minutes, so the flavors can develop, then serve hot!

Spaghetti Squash with Bacon Blue Cheese

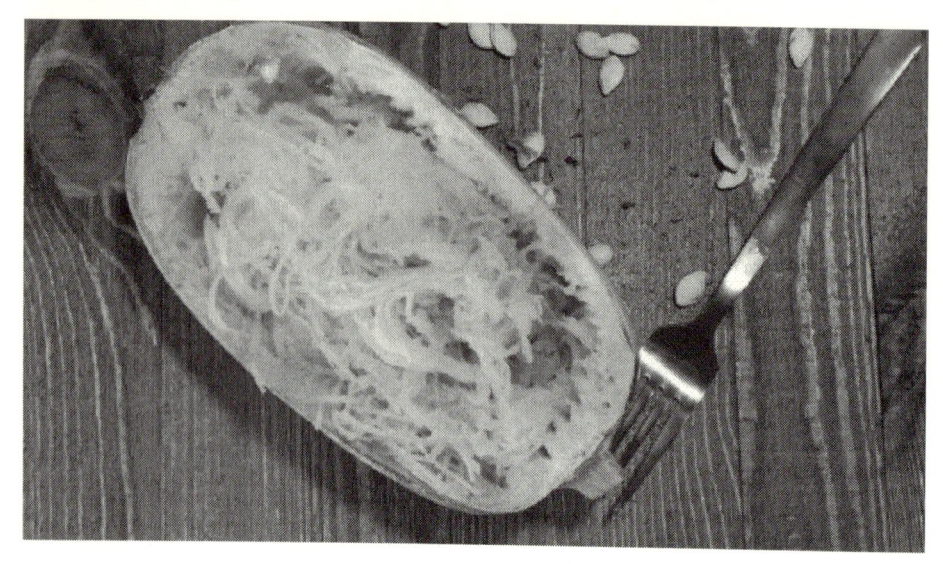

Nutrition
Calories per serving: 339
Carbohydrates: 21 grams
Fat: 24 grams
Fiber: 1 gram
Protein: 13.5 grams

Ingredients

¼ c. sour cream
1 sm. spaghetti squash
1 tbsp. extra virgin olive oil
1 clove garlic, minced
2 c. baby spinach
2 tbsp. bleu cheese crumbles
4 slices bacon, chopped
4 oz. mushrooms, sliced
Salt and pepper to taste

Directions

1. Preheat the oven to 400 degrees Fahrenheit and line a baking sheet with foil.
2. Using a very sharp knife, cut your spaghetti squash in half lengthwise and use a spoon to hollow out the loose strings and seeds in the center.
3. Coat the inside of the squash with olive oil, then generously sprinkle with salt and pepper.
4. Bake for about 45 minutes, then scrape the insides out of the squash and into a large bowl. Set aside and place the shells back on the baking sheet.
5. In a large skillet, cook your bacon over minute high heat and drain over paper towels.
6. Cook mushrooms and garlic in the skillet for four to five minutes, then stir the bacon and the spinach into the pan until the spinach is wilted, about two or three minutes.
7. Spoon the mixture over the squash and add the sour cream, salt, and pepper to the bowl, stirring to evenly combine.
8. Spoon the mixture into the shells, top with 1 tablespoon of bleu cheese and bake for four to five minutes, until the cheese has heated through.

Spinach Artichoke Chicken

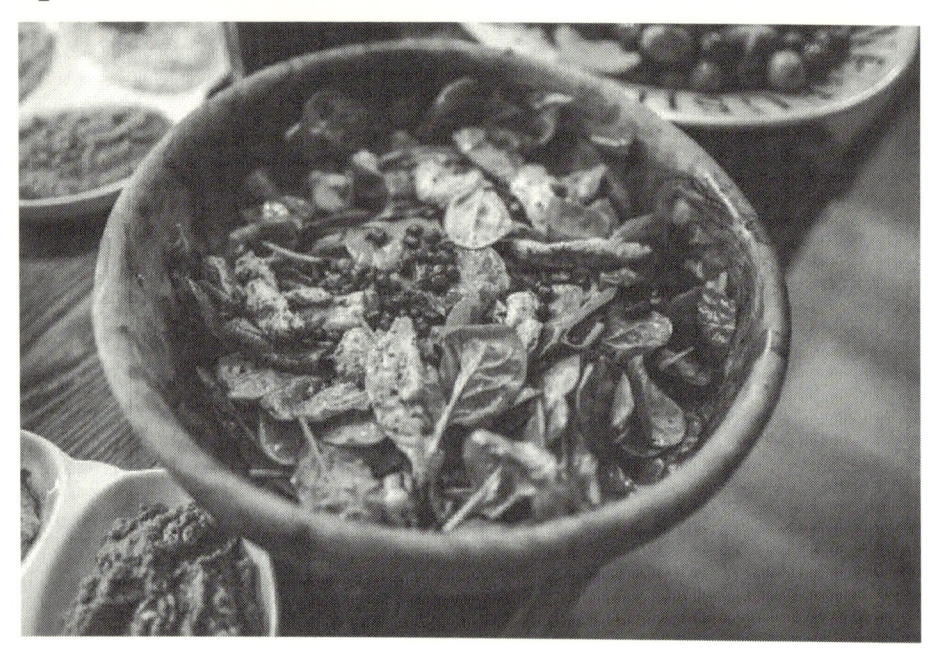

Nutrition
Calories per serving: 554
Carbohydrates: 5 grams
Fat: 33 grams
Fiber: 1 gram
Protein: 56 grams

Ingredients

¼ c. parmesan cheese, shredded
¼ c. mayonnaise
½ tsp. garlic powder
½ tsp. salt
½ c. mozzarella cheese, shredded
1 tbsp. extra virgin olive oil
4 oz. cream cheese, softened
5 oz. spinach, frozen & drained
8 oz. chicken breasts, boneless & skinless

14 oz. quartered artichoke hearts, drained & chopped
Salt and pepper to taste

Directions
1. Preheat the oven to 375 degrees Fahrenheit.
2. Once you are certain the moisture has been purged from your spinach, add it into a medium-sized mixing bowl with cream cheese, parmesan cheese, artichoke hearts, garlic powder, mayonnaise, and salt. Stir to completely combine and set it aside.
3. Pound out the chicken breasts until they're a little less than an inch thick and then season on both sides with salt and pepper.
4. Heat olive oil in a skillet over medium heat. Cook the chicken breasts for about two to three minutes per side, until a golden crust forms on both sides.
5. In a large baking dish, layer the chicken breasts and the spinach artichoke mixture. Bake for 20 to 22 minutes, until the chicken is cooked completely through. The juices should run clear and the internal temperature should be 165 degrees Fahrenheit.
6. Top the breasts with mozzarella cheese, then pop back into the oven until the cheese is melted.
7. Serve hot!

Korean Beef over Cauliflower Rice

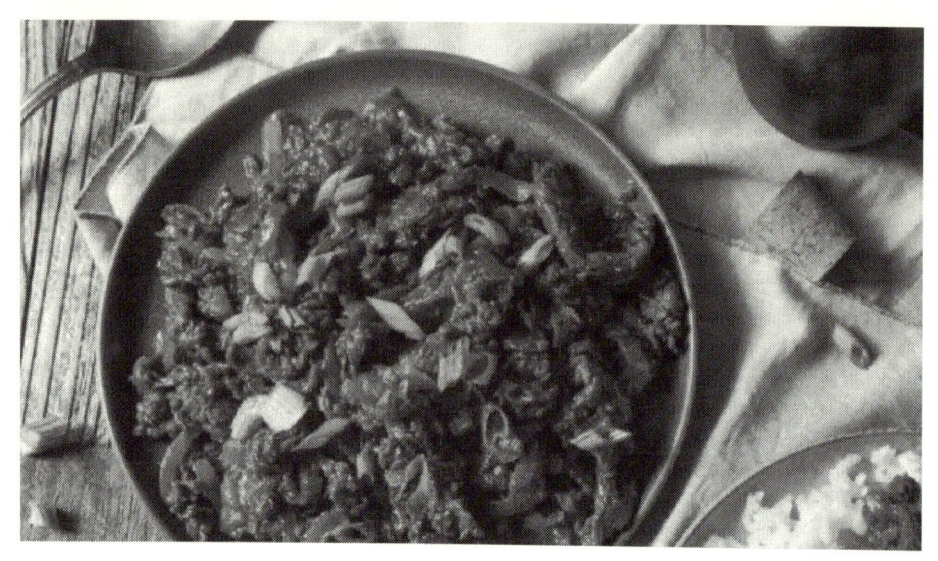

Nutrition
Calories per serving: 297
Carbohydrates: 9 grams
Fat: 19.1 grams
Fiber: 2 grams
Protein: 22 grams

Ingredients

¼ c. soy sauce
¼ tsp. ground black pepper
¼ tsp. ground ginger
1 lb. ground beef
1 tbsp. coconut sugar
1 med. green onion, chopped
1 tbsp. sesame seeds
2 tsp. sesame oil
2 c. cauliflower rice
3 cloves garlic, minced

Directions

1. In a large skillet over medium heat, warm the sesame oil.
2. Brown the beef and the minced garlic for about 5 to 7 minutes, or until completely cooked through.
3. Add the soy sauce, ginger, coconut sugar, and black pepper into a small bowl and whisk until completely combined.
4. Pour the sauce over the beef and stir it completely. Allow to simmer for about three minutes so the sauce can thicken.
5. Serve over cauliflower rice, topped with sesame seeds and green onions.

CHAPTER 12: KETO SNACK RECIPES

Parmesan Zucchini Fries

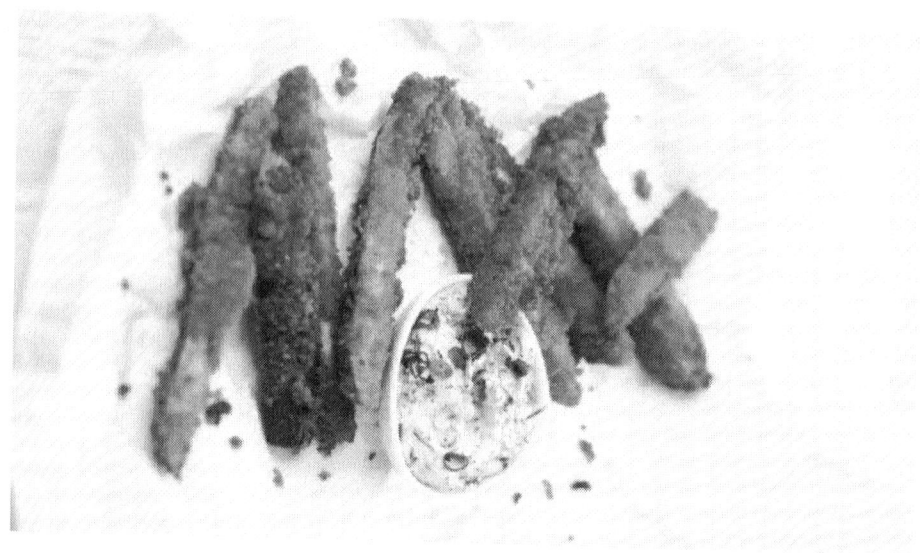

Nutrition
Calories per serving: 142
Carbohydrates: 10 grams
Fat: 7 grams
Fiber: 3 grams
Protein: 12 grams

Ingredients

½ tsp. ground black pepper
¾ c. parmesan cheese, grated
1 tbsp. mixed herbs, dried
1 tsp. paprika
1 ½ tsp. garlic powder
2 lg. eggs
2 lbs. zucchini, cut into french-fry shapes

Directions
1. Preheat the oven to 425 degrees Fahrenheit and line a baking pan with foil, then grease it with cooking spray.
2. In a shallow dish, whisk the eggs completely. In another shallow dish, combine the herbs, garlic powder, pepper, parmesan cheese, and paprika and mix well.
3. Dip your zucchini fries into the eggs in batches and shake each one to remove the excess egg.
4. Then dip the zucchini pieces into the parmesan mixture, rolling to coat completely.
5. Place in an even layer on a baking sheet.
6. Bake for 30 to 35 minutes, turning them once halfway through, until golden and crisp.
7. Serve hot and crispy!

Zesty Ranch Cauliflower Crisps

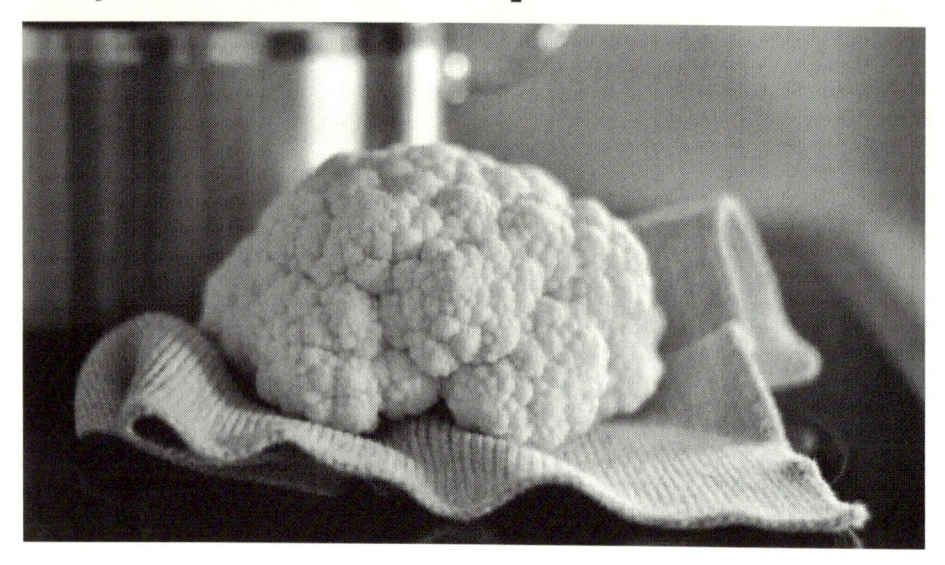

Nutrition
Calories per serving: 29
Carbohydrates: 1 gram
Fat: 1.5 grams
Fiber: <1 gram
Protein: 2.5 grams

Ingredients

1 lg. egg
1 tbsp. dry ranch salad dressing mix
1 c. parmesan cheese, shredded
12 oz. frozen cauliflower, riced
Cayenne pepper to taste

Directions
1. In a microwave-safe bowl, cover the frozen riced cauliflower, cover, and heat for 3 to 4 minutes.
2. Allow to cool enough to handle, then place the cauliflower in a kitchen towel or cheesecloth and strain completely.

3. Preheat the oven to 425 degrees Fahrenheit and line a baking sheet with parchment paper.
4. In the bowl with the cauliflower, combine the ranch mix, the egg, and the cayenne and mix completely. Stir the parmesan cheese into the mix and stir until everything is completely mixed.
5. Place the mix in small, flat dollops on the baking sheet, making sure that the pieces are all evenly-sized and thin. The thinner your mixture, the crispier your cracker will be.
6. Bake for 10 minutes, flip, then bake for another 10 minutes. Allow the crackers to cool on a wire rack completely, then enjoy!

Peanut Butter Bars

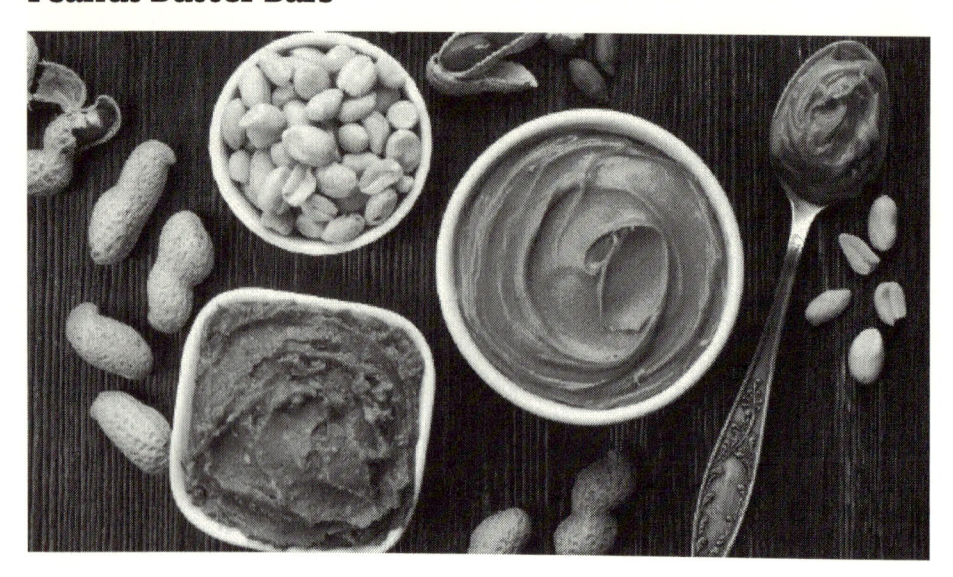

Nutrition
Calories per serving: 182
Carbohydrates: 25 grams
Fat: 14 grams
Fiber: <1 gram
Protein: 3.5 grams

Ingredients

½ c. butter
½ c. creamy peanut butter
1 c. powdered erythritol sweetener
1 c. keto graham cracker crumbs
1 c. sugar-free dark chocolate chips
2 tbsp. creamy peanut butter

Directions

1. Line an 8-inch square baking pan with parchment paper lining the bottom and sides.
2. Melt the butter and then add powdered sweetener, crumbs, and the ½ cup of peanut butter. Mix until com-

pletely combined then press the mixture evenly into the bottom of the prepared pan.
3. In a small, microwave-safe bowl, heat the 2 tablespoons of peanut butter and the chocolate chips at 20-second intervals for about 2 minutes, or until you can mix them smoothly together.
4. Pour the mixture over the mix in the baking pan and spread it evenly with a spatula or spoon.
5. Refrigerate for about 30 minutes, then score the top with cut lines. This will keep the chocolate from cracking when you cut your bars.
6. Place them back in the refrigerator until firm (about 30 more minutes), then cut and serve!

Lemon Poppy Seed Muffins

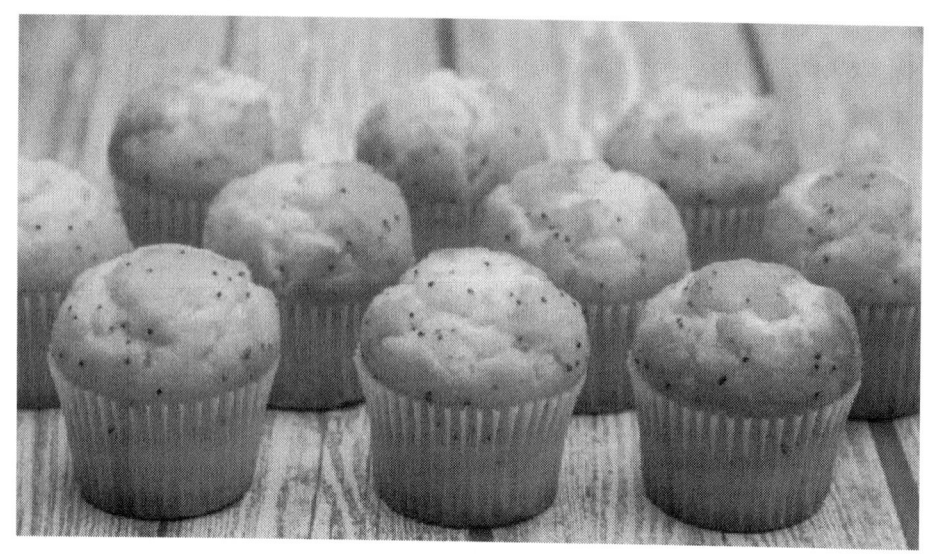

Nutrition
Calories per serving: 116
Carbohydrates: 10 grams
Fat: 11 grams
Fiber: <1 gram
Protein: 4 grams

Ingredients

⅓ c. sugar-free sweetener of your choice
¼ c. almond flour
¼ c. coconut flour
¼ tsp. xanthan gum
½ tsp. vanilla extract
½ tsp. baking powder
½ tsp. salt
1 tbsp. poppy seeds
1 lemon, zested
2 tbsp. sour cream
2 tbsp. heavy whipping cream
3 lg. eggs

3 tbsp. butter

Directions
1. Preheat the oven to 350 degrees Fahrenheit and grease a muffin tin with non-stick spray or with muffin liners.
2. In a large bowl, combine the flours, seeds, zest, sweetener, baking powder, salt, and xanthan gum and stir completely.
3. In another bowl, beat the eggs with an electric mixer until they are fluffy. Beat the butter, vanilla, and sour cream into the eggs. Then add the flour mixture. Cream the ingredients slowly until they're thick and smooth.
4. Pour the batter into the tins, then bake until the tops are golden, about 15 to 20 minutes.

CHAPTER 13: KETO DESSERT RECIPES

Chewy Chocolate Cookies

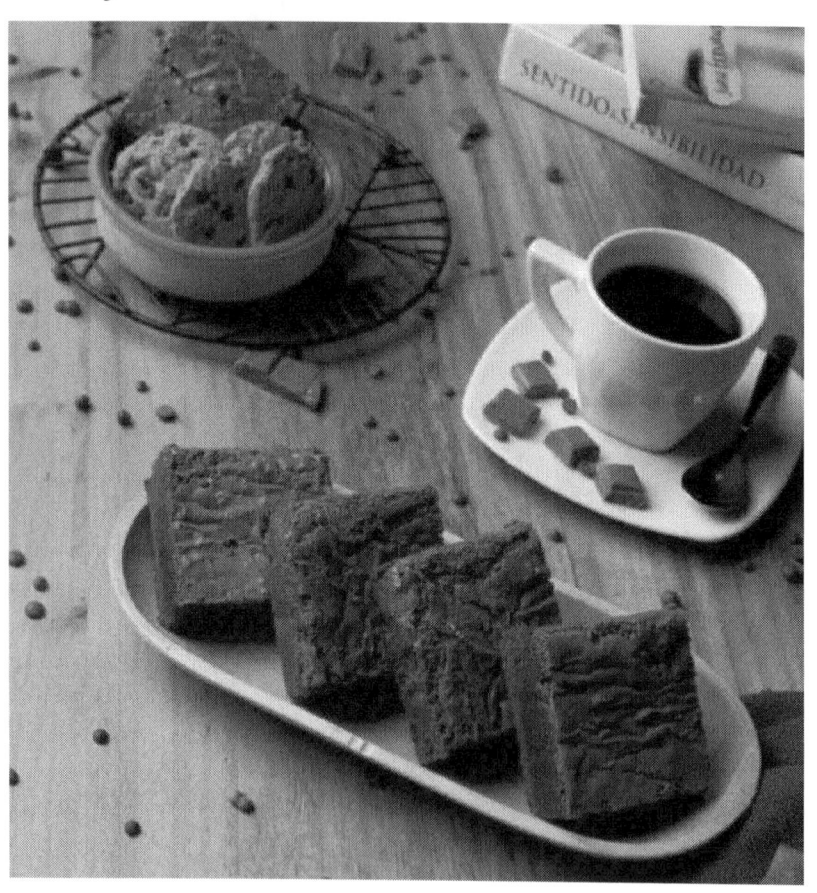

Nutrition
Calories per serving: 173
Carbohydrates: 13 grams
Fat: 16 grams
Fiber: 2 grams
Protein: 5 grams
Ingredients

½ c. sugar-free sweetener of choice
⅓ c. cocoa powder, unsweetened & sifted
1 tsp. vanilla extract
1 pinch salt
1 ½ c. almond butter
2 lg. eggs

Directions
1. Preheat the oven to 350 degrees Fahrenheit and line a baking pan with parchment paper.
2. In a food processor, combine the eggs, almond butter, vanilla extract, cocoa powder, and salt. Pulse until a dough forms.
3. Roll the dough into 1-inch balls and place them on the baking sheet, pressing down on the tops of each with a fork twice to make a crisscross pattern on them.
4. Bake until the edges are firm, about 12 minutes. Allow to cool for a minute or so before transferring to a wire rack to cool completely.
5. Enjoy!

Berry Cheesecake Bars

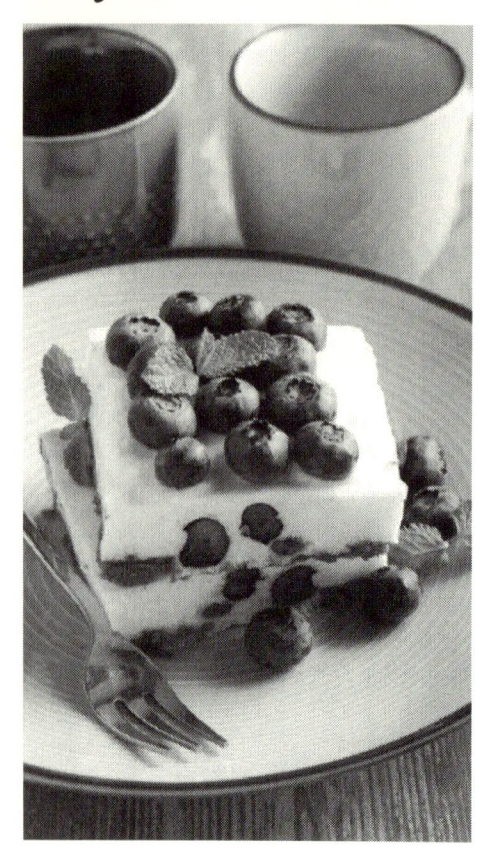

Nutrition
Calories per serving: 155
Carbohydrates: 11 grams
Fat: 14 grams
Fiber: 1 gram
Protein: 3 grams
Ingredients

For the crust:

¼ tsp. ground nutmeg
1 c. pecans
1 tsp. sugar-free sweetener

1 tsp. ground cinnamon
2 tbsp. melted butter

For the filling:

¼ c. almond milk, unsweetened
¼ c. sour cream
½ tsp. vanilla extract
½ c. sugar-free sweetener
1 tbsp. butter, melted
1 lg. egg
12 oz. cream cheese

For the topping:

1 c. frozen mixed berries
1 tbsp. sugar-free sweetener

Directions
1. Preheat the oven to 350 degrees Fahrenheit and line a baking pan with parchment paper.
2. In a food processor, pulse the pecans until finely chopped. Add the sweetener, cinnamon, and nutmeg, then process for a few seconds more.
3. Pour the mixture into a bowl and combine with the melted butter.
4. Once mixed, press the mixture into the bottom of a baking dish to form the crust.
5. In a large bowl, beat the egg with an electric mixture until it's fluffy. Mix one ounce of cream cheese into the bowl at a time and beat until smooth. Add the sweetener, vanilla extract, sour cream, and the almond milk. Beat them together until the mixture is completely smooth, then pour the filling over the crust.
6. Bake for about 35 minutes.
7. While the bars are baking, heat a small pot over medium heat and add the mixed berries and sweetener to

it. Bring them to a simmer and allow to cook for about 5 minutes. Stir the berries and crush them lightly with a spoon so a liquid begins to form in the pot, then simmer for another 10 minutes.
8. Allow the bars to cool for about 1 hour, then top with the berry sauce.
9. Serve!

Coconut Lime Bars

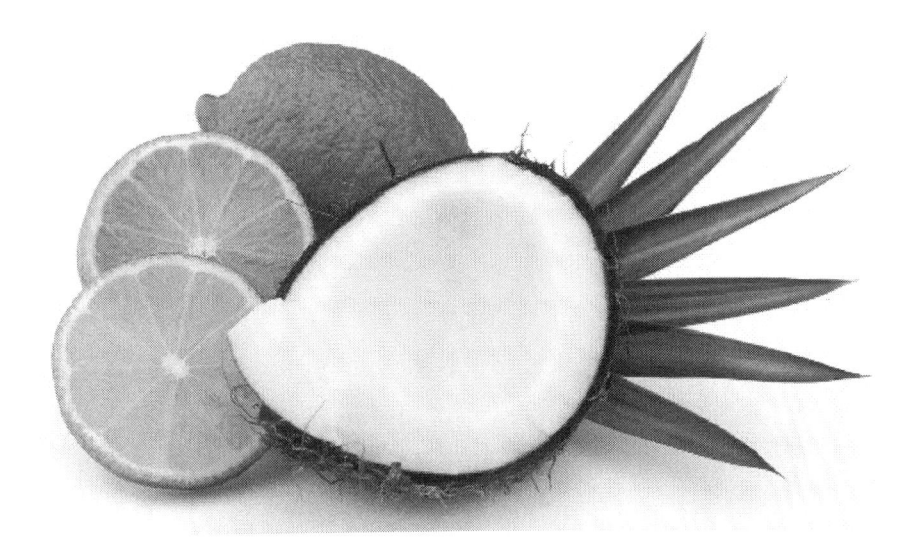

Nutrition
Calories per serving: 160
Carbohydrates: 18 grams
Fat: 14 grams
Fiber: 2 grams
Protein: 5 grams

Ingredients

For the crust:

¼ tsp. salt
½ c. sugar-free sweetener
1 c. almond flour, finely ground
1 tsp. lime zest
2 tbsp. coconut flour
3 tbsp. butter, softened

For the filling:

½ c. coconut milk
½ c. sugar-free sweetener

1 c. lime juice
1 tbsp. butter
1 tsp. lime zest
5 lg. eggs, beaten

For the topping:

½ tbsp. lime zest
2 tbsp. shredded coconut, unsweetened

Directions

1. Preheat the oven to 350 degrees Fahrenheit and grease a square baking dish.
2. In a large bowl, combine the almond flour, coconut flour, sweetener, lime zest, and salt. Mix and cut in the butter with a fork until combined and there are no lumps. Press the crust mixture into the baking dish until it's even.
3. Bake for 10 to 15 minutes, then set aside.
4. In a medium saucepan over medium heat, combine the coconut milk, sweetener, lime juice, coconut milk, and butter. Mix until the sweetener is completely dissolved, then add the beaten eggs a little bit at a time until the mixture is foamy and airy and just starting to thicken, about 5 to 10 minutes.
5. Pour the filling into the crust and bake for about 10 to 15 minutes to set the filling all the way through.
6. Toast the shredded coconut in a small skillet until just lightly browned, then top the bars with it.
7. Allow the bars to cool, slice, and serve cold!

Strawberry Ice Cream

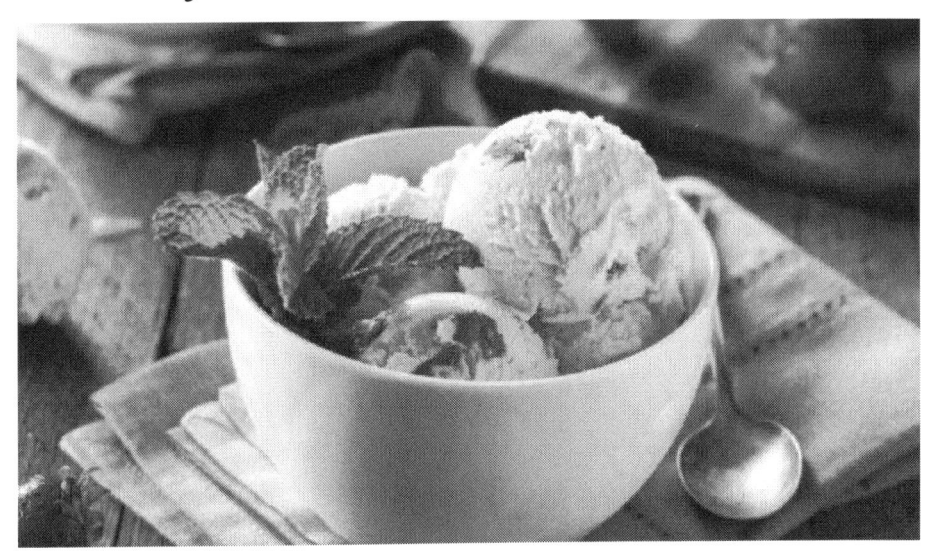

Nutrition
Calories per serving: 264
Carbohydrates: 19 grams
Fat: 28 grams
Fiber: <1 gram
Protein: grams

Ingredients

½ tsp. vodka
½ c. water
⅔ c. sugar-free sweetener
1 tsp. lemon juice
1 pinch salt
2 ½ c. heavy whipping cream
2 tsp. vanilla extract
5 strawberries, hulled

Directions
1. Puree the strawberries in the food processor until smooth.

2. Whisk the puree, cream, sweetener, water, vanilla, vodka, and salt in a bowl.
3. Once completely mixed, pour the mixture into the ice cream maker.
4. Process the ice cream to manufacturer instructions, transfer into a freezer-safe container, and freeze!
5. If you don't have an ice cream maker, pour the mix into a loaf pan, press some plastic wrap down onto the entire surface of the ice cream, then freeze to set!

Conclusion

Thank you for making it through to the end of *Keto for Cancer: A Practical Guide to a Healthful and Natural Approach to Stopping and Slowing Cancer Growth with Metabolic Recovery*, I hope the information in this book has given you some strength and power to get through what is undoubtedly a difficult time for you and your family.

In this book, you've learned everything from the very basics of what cancer is, how it's formed, how it spreads, and what things might feed into it, helping it to spread faster throughout your body. You've learned about the things that can commonly cause issues for those who turn to keto for the answers about their illnesses, and you've learned about all the most effective ways to turn things around for the best possible outcome.

I've walked you through the explanations about how food is processed in the body, what happens to those excess sugars, how you can cut those down, and how those could relate to cancer or other illness. I've explained that following the advice and treatment of your doctor always comes first, and I've given you details about how to incorporate your efforts in the kitchen with the doctor's efforts to keep you feeling your best.

Now that you understand all of the things that are at play here and now that you know of all the ways in which you can safeguard your own physical health, it's time to put what you know to work for you. It's time to test out all that's been said here and make a plan to use this information throughout your treatment.

Always stay in contact with your doctor about the things you're planning on changing in your regimen when you're getting consistent treatment, regardless of the illness. The more your doctor knows about the approach you're taking when you're not with your doctor, the better equipped they are to help you to achieve the best possible results in your treatment.

Remember that your doctor only sees you during your appointments, so they're only aware of the things that you tell them when you see them. Make sure you're as clear with your doctor as possible about your concerns, your efforts, what you know, what you don't know, and you will find that your doctor can help you much more readily that way. In some cases, you might find that your doctor has corrections to make in the assumptions you have, the conclusions you've reached, or the methods that you've chosen. Make sure you're receptive to those changes, but be certain to ask for explanations.

The more educated you are about the nature of your treatment, the reasons for certain aspects of it, and the effects of everything that's in play, it can help you to take ownership of your treatment plan. It can help you to more readily take responsibility for certain aspects of it and make sure that everything is going along as well as it should be at each and every stage of the process. If you're having trouble with how something might work or with applying it in your life, don't be afraid to ask questions. Asking those questions gets information that will undoubtedly come in handy during some point or another in your life.

Now that you've read all of this and you've started to educate yourself on the nature of the illness at hand, you're ready to move forward and put your plans into action. Between you and your doctor, you will be able to devise a treatment plan that is right for you and for your family. There is no doubt in my mind that the treatment will be difficult, but the road ahead is clear and you have the strength within you to traverse it.

Thank you very much for purchasing and reading *Keto for Cancer: A Practical Guide to a Healthful and Natural Approach to Stop-*

ping and Slowing Cancer Growth with Metabolic Recovery and I hope very much that you have found some information and some tips in this book that can help you. If you have enjoyed this book, if you've learned something from it, or if you've found anything helpful or useful in this book, please do leave an Amazon review for it.

I strive to bring my readers the best possible content on the subjects that are in-demand and your reviews help me to make the necessary adjustments to do just that. Thank you once again and best of luck to you and your family on the road ahead.

Resources

Ketogenic Diets and Cancer: Emerging Evidence. (n.d.), from https://www.ncbi.nlm.nih.gov/pmc/articles/PMC6375425/

Mitochondrial dysfunction in cancer. - PubMed - NCBI. (n.d.). Retrieved from https://www.ncbi.nlm.nih.gov/m/pubmed/26327844/

The CUP Foundation
https://cupfoundjo.org/what-is-cup/frequently-asked-questions-about-cancer

The American Cancer Society
https://www.cancer.org/cancer/cancer-basics/questions-people-ask-about-cancer.html

The National Cancer Institute:
https://www.cancer.gov/about-cancer/understanding/statistics

US National Library of Medicine, National Institutes of Health
https://www.ncbi.nlm.nih.gov/pmc/articles/PMC3873478/

Elsevier Gynecologic Oncology
https://www.sciencedirect.com/science/article/abs/pii/S0090825815300573

The books I referenced are:

Hoffman, V. (n.d.). Ketogenic Instant Pot Cookbook: The Best 100 Keto Instant Pot Recipes To Lose Weight and Being Healthy! - Kindle edition by Virginia Hoffman. Cookbooks, Food & Wine Kindle eBooks @ Amazon.com. Retrieved from https://www.amazon.com/Ketogenic-Instant-Pot-Cookbook-Recipes-ebook/dp/B079SP375M

Hoffman, H. (n.d.). Ketogenic Diet: Rapid Weight Loss Snacks VOLUME 1: Lose Up To 30 Lbs. In 30 Days by Henry

Brooke. Retrieved from https://www.goodreads.com/book/show/27134477-ketogenic-diet

Kaplan, J. (n.d.). Ketogenic Diet: James Kaplan: 9781523333974. Retrieved from https://www.bookdepository.com/Ketogenic-Diet-James-Kaplan/9781523333974

Keto for Cancer: Ketogenic Metabolic Therapy as a Targeted Nutritional Strategy: 9781603587013: Medicine & Health Science Books @ Amazon.com. (n.d.). Retrieved fr
https://www.amazon.com/Keto-Cancer-Ketogenic-Metabolic-Nutritional/dp/1603587012

Made in the USA
Middletown, DE
23 April 2023